PIGS: WELFARE IN PRACTICE

PIGS: WELFARE IN PRACTICE

Edited by Irene Camerlink

Series Editor: Xavier Manteca Vilanova

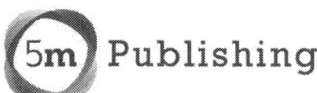

5m Publishing

Published by
5m Publishing Ltd,
Benchmark House,
8 Smithy Wood Drive,
Sheffield, S35 1QN, UK
Tel: +44 (0) 1234 81 81 80
www.5mpublishing.com

A Catalogue record for this book is available from the British Library

ISBN 9781789181050

Book layout by KSPM, 8 Wood Road, Codsall, Wolverhampton, WV8 1DB
Printed by Hobbs The Printers Ltd, Totton, Hampshire

Pig illustrations by Henry Cruickshank
Other photos and illustrations as indicated in the text

Contents

Contributors

Prof Rita Albernaz-Goncalves, Instituto Federal de Educação, Ciência e Tecnologia Catarinense, Santa Rosa do Sul, Brazil

Dr Mabel Aworh-Ajumobi, Department of Veterinary & Pests Control Services, Federal Ministry of Agriculture & Rural Development, Abuja, Nigeria

Dr Emma M. Baxter, Animal Behaviour & Welfare, Animal and Veterinary Sciences Research Group, Scotland's Rural College (SRUC), Edinburgh, UK

Prof Elodie F. Briefer, Behavioural Ecology Group, Section for Ecology & Evolution, Department of Biology, University of Copenhagen, Copenhagen, Denmark

Dr Jennifer Brown, Prairie Swine Centre, Saskatoon, Canada

Dr Irene Camerlink, Institute of Genetics and Animal Breeding, Polish Academy of Sciences, Jastrzebiec, Poland

Maria Chen, Animal Welfare Program, Faculty of Land and Food Systems, University of British Columbia, Vancouver, Canada

Dr Antoni Dalmau, IRTA, Animal Welfare Program, Monells, Spain

Dr Rick B. D'Eath, Animal Behaviour & Welfare, Animal and Veterinary Sciences Research Group, Scotland's Rural College (SRUC), Edinburgh, UK

Dr Nicolas Devillers, Agriculture and Agri-Food Canada, Sherbrooke Research and Development Centre, Sherbrooke, Canada

Dr Mette S. Herskin, Department of Animal Science, Aarhus University, Tjele, Denmark

Prof Paul H. Hemsworth, Animal Welfare Science Centre, Faculty of Veterinary and Agricultural Sciences, University of Melbourne, Parkville, VIC, Australia

Prof Maria José Hötzel, Laboratório de Etologia Aplicada e Bem-Estar Animal, Departamento de Zootecnia e Desenvolvimento Rural, Universidade Federal de Santa Catarina, Florianópolis, Brazil

Dr Sarah Ison, World Animal Protection, London, UK

Prof Marina von Keyserlingk, Animal Welfare Program, Faculty of Land and Food Systems, University of British Columbia, Vancouver, Canada

Cecilie Kobek-Kjeldager, Department of Animal Science, Aarhus University, Tjele, Denmark

Dr Hanne Kongsted, Department of Animal Science, Aarhus University, Tjele, Denmark

Dr Mona Lilian Vestbjerg Larsen, Department of Animal Science, Aarhus University, Tjele, Denmark

Prof Alistair B. Lawrence, Animal Behaviour & Welfare, Animal and Veterinary Sciences Research Group, Scotland's Rural College (SRUC), Edinburgh, UK

Dr Lisette M. C. Leliveld, Institute of Behavioural Physiology, Leibniz Institute for Farm Animal Biology (FBN), Dummerstorf, Germany

Prof Jeremy N. Marchant-Forde, USDA Agricultural Research Service, Livestock Behavior Research Unit, West Lafayette, USA

Dr Martyna M. Małopolska, Department of Pig Breeding, National Research Institute of Animal Production, Balice near Kraków, Poland

Prof John J. McGlone, Animal and Food Sciences, Texas Tech University, Lubbock, USA

Dr Maciej Oczak, Precision Livestock Farming Hub (PLF-Hub) / Institute of Animal Welfare Science, University of Veterinary Medicine, Vienna, Austria

Dr Winfried Otten, Institute of Behavioural Physiology, Leibniz Institute for Farm Animal Biology (FBN), Dummerstorf, Germany

Dr Monique D. Pairis-Garcia, Global Production Animal Welfare, Department of Population Health and Pathobiology, North Carolina State University College of Veterinary Medicine, Raleigh, USA

Dr Rachel S. E. Peden, Animal Behaviour & Welfare, Animal and Veterinary Sciences Research Group, Scotland's Rural College (SRUC), Edinburgh, UK

Prof Lene Juul Pedersen, Department of Animal Science, Aarhus University, Tjele, Denmark

Prof Clive J. C. Phillips, Centre for Animal Welfare and Ethics, School of Veterinary Science, University of Queensland, Gatton, Australia

Prof Jean-Loup Rault, Institute of Animal Welfare Science, University of Veterinary Medicine, Vienna, Austria

Prof Lotta Rydhmer, Department of Animal Breeding and Genetics, Swedish University of Agricultural Sciences, Uppsala, Sweden

Dr Yolande Seddon, Department of Large Animal Clinical Sciences, Western College of Veterinary Medicine, University of Saskatchewan, Saskatchewan, Canada

Jeremy M. Skuse, Animal Welfare Science Centre, Faculty of Veterinary and Agricultural Sciences, University of Melbourne, Parkville, VIC, Australia

Rebecca Sommerville, Behaviour By Becca, London, UK

Dr Marek Špinka, Department of Ethology and Companion Animal Science, Faculty of Agrobiology, Food and Natural Resources, Czech University of Life Sciences, Prague, Czechia

Dr Hans A. M. Spoolder, Wageningen Livestock Research, Wageningen, the Netherlands

Prof John Strak, Food Economics, School of Biosciences, University of Nottingham, UK

Dr Céline Tallet, INRAE, Agrocampus Ouest, PEGASE, Saint-Gilles, France

Dr Dayane Lemos Teixeira, Instituto de Ciencias Agronómicas y Veterinarias, Universidad de O'Higgins, San Fernando, Chile

Dr Simon P. Turner, Animal Behaviour & Welfare, Animal and Veterinary Sciences Research Group, Scotland's Rural College (SRUC), Edinburgh, UK

Dr Ryszard Tuz, Department of Swine and Small Animal Breeding, University of Agriculture in Kraków, Kraków, Poland

Dr Heleen A. van de Weerd, Cerebrus Associates Ltd., Newark, UK

Dr Nienke van Staaveren, Department of Animal Biosciences, University of Guelph, Guelph, Canada

Prof Anna Valros, Research Centre for Animal Welfare, Department of Production Animal Medicine, Faculty of Veterinary Medicine, University of Helsinki, Finland

Dr Antonio Velarde Calvo, IRTA, Animal Welfare Program, Monells, Spain

Dr Megan Verdon, Tasmanian Institute of Agriculture, University of Tasmania, Tasmania, Australia

Prof Françoise Wemelsfelder, Animal Behaviour & Welfare, Animal and Veterinary Sciences Research Group, Scotland's Rural College (SRUC), Edinburgh, UK

Dr Maria Cristina Yunes, Laboratório de Etologia Aplicada e Bem-Estar Animal, Departamento de Zootecnia e Desenvolvimento Rural, Universidade Federal de Santa Catarina, Florianópolis, Brazil

Foreword

Pig welfare is a very active area of research and the amount of scientific information that is published every year can be truly overwhelming. This book provides an excellent summary of our current knowledge of pig welfare using a concise, easy-to-understand language and a very practical approach that will be very useful for veterinarians, animal scientist and pig producers, among others.

The book is divided into four sections. The first, Understanding pig welfare, introduces the concept of animal welfare and gives an overview of the main issues related to pig welfare in different parts of the world. The second, Making the business case for animal welfare, discusses the economic benefits of improving animal welfare on pig farms and includes three examples of cost–benefit analysis. The third, Assessing animal welfare, covers a selection of welfare indicators as well as qualitative behaviour assessment, welfare assessment methods, welfare apps and the use of Precision Livestock Farming to identify welfare risks. The fourth, What can you do to improve animal welfare?, discusses the main strategies available to improve pig welfare on farm. In each section, the authors have done an excellent job at providing both a review of the fundamental aspects of pig welfare together with a set of practical recommendations on how to perform a cost–benefit analysis of animal welfare, how to assess the welfare of pigs and how to design a stepwise action plan to improving animal welfare on pig farms.

The book has been written by an impressive team of more than 40 contributors led by Dr Irene Camerlink. The list of authors includes most of the key experts in the field from around the world, which ensures that different production conditions are taken into account and gives the book a truly global approach.

I truly hope that this book will be very useful for those working in pig production and will make a significant contribution to the improvement of pig welfare.

Professor Xavier Manteca

Series Editor

Farm Animal Welfare Education Centre (FAWEC)

School of Veterinary Science

Universitat Autònoma de Barcelona, Spain

Introduction

Animal welfare has become in many countries an integral part of animal husbandry. Whereas in some parts of the world animal welfare is considered because of moral concern, for cultural reasons or its link to productivity, in other parts, it has mainly been enforced by legislation, encouraged through assurance schemes or demanded by retailers. The latter set of drivers has put pressure on many producers worldwide as they need to adjust their systems to proscribed requirements. This initially may seem to disadvantage their market position compared to countries where animal welfare is not as much part of the political agenda or societal debate. Animal welfare is, however, much more than just the guidelines set by policymakers. In fact, improving animal welfare can be very favourable for productivity when integrated well in farm management. As most animal welfare issues are multifactorial, such as tail biting, case-to-case solutions may be needed. As there are generally no farm advisors for welfare, like there are veterinarians and farm advisors for nutrition and genetics, this handbook gives some practical advice on how you can improve the welfare of your pigs yourself.

About this book

This book is part of a series of short, practical books on the welfare of farmed animals. The series covers what is currently known about the welfare requirements of specific animal species and how to put this into practice. Its aim is to provide people in different countries with a tool to improve animal welfare through scientifically based information presented in a concise, easy to understand way. *Pigs: Welfare in Practice* focuses on pigs kept for commercial husbandry. The book is aimed at farmers, stockworkers and animal handlers, and additionally as a reference for smallholders, animal scientists and agricultural students.

The chapters in this book are written by esteemed researchers from all over the world. Most have studied pig behaviour, welfare and production for many years whereas some share their knowledge of economics. Besides their role as scientist they actively engage in knowledge exchange by advising farmers and other stakeholders.

In Chapter 1 the concept of animal welfare is explained, along with the specific requirements of pigs kept for production purposes. The current state of pig welfare on a global scale is described, with the main developments in production and legislation. Chapter 2 gives examples of how animal welfare can contribute to increased profitability and how you can assess the costs and benefits of improving welfare. Chapter 3 outlines the main methods of assessing the welfare of pigs. This will give insight on how your animals are doing. Specific attention is given to so-called iceberg indicators. These can give an indication of underlying welfare beyond the key observable trait. In Chapter 4 suggestions are given for how you can improve the welfare of pigs, organized by production phase.

How to use this book

At the end of each chapter there is a section offering advice on applying the information to your own pig herd. Look for the 📝 symbol, which indicates farm assessment sections. At end of the book, in the appendices, you will find the scoring sheets. Want to use them again? The blank forms can be downloaded from the book's companion webpage (https://www.5mbooks.com/pigs-welfare-in-practice).

The suggestions given in this book are based on repeated scientific studies with most methods having been tested under commercial conditions. This is, however, no guarantee that a certain strategy will be effective on every farm, in every situation. Please be cautious with making changes in the management and monitor the animals closely. Consult with the veterinarian if required.

CHAPTER 1

Understanding pig welfare

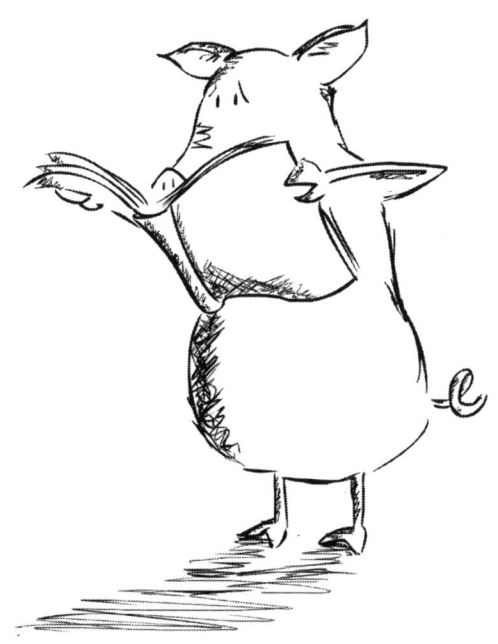

1.1 Good welfare, more than just being healthy

MAREK ŠPINKA

Animal welfare may be simply defined as the quality of life that an animal has in its real conditions. There are three main factors that compose the quality of life, in other words, those that matter to the animal (Figure 1.1):

1. its biological functioning: the state of being fit and healthy

2. its behavioural coping: successful engagement with the outside world

3. its subjective feelings: experience of positive as opposed to negative affective states.

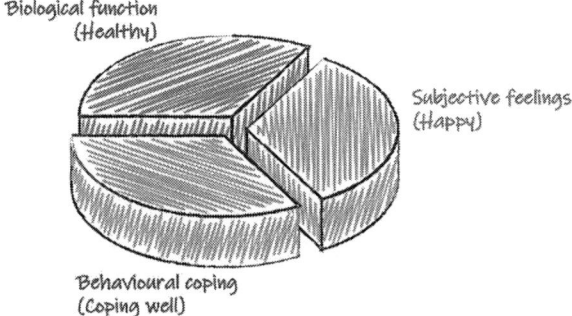

Figure 1.1 The main attributes that determine animal welfare.
Illustration: I. Camerlink.

Wild living animals have been endowed with species-specific physiological, behavioural and psychological capabilities through the process of natural selection. These include, on the one hand, negative mechanisms such as pain or fever to cope with injury and infection, aggressive behaviour to overcome competitors or fear emotion to avoid predators. On the other hand, there are positive mechanisms, such as a balanced metabolism for the utilization of nutrients, social behaviour to maintain company or the contentment emotion to reward success. In farm animals, such as the pig, all the mechanisms of physiological, behavioural and psychological functioning of the wild ancestor species are maintained, although some of them have been quantitatively strengthened or diminished through the processes of domestication and selective breeding. Therefore, for a domestic pig to have a good quality of life, it needs to live in an environment that promotes positive physiological, behavioural and mental functioning and does not trigger negative mechanisms.

Ethically, there is wide agreement that when humans keep animals in captivity, they become responsible for their quality of life. Thus we – the human society – should provide farm animals with living conditions that are conducive to good welfare. Practically, it is the farmers that set up and run the environment for livestock, but their decisions are affected by societal conditions, such as consumer demand, the economic situation, legislation and public opinion. Thus, the concept of animal welfare needs to be understood both from the point of view of farmer and from the point of view of the society at large.

Farmers are motivated to provide good care of their animals and keep them healthy in order to support their high performance. For practically minded farmers, the question thus arises: Why is the extra term 'animal welfare' needed anyway? Therefore, it is useful to clarify the relationships and differences between animal performance, animal health and animal welfare.

Performance and health are closely related in pigs. Poor health undermines the capacity for growth and reproduction. At the same time, prolific reproduction and fast growth puts pressure on health and welfare. In past decades, breeding programmes emphasized performance traits and consequently the current genotypes of pigs channel resources into production rather than into maintenance and health, putting the animals under reproductive and metabolic strain and making them more susceptible to illness and injury. Therefore, high producing pigs need intense and highly skilled monitoring, support and intervention, if they are to live a healthy life.

The relationship between pig health and pig welfare is that of inclusion – pig welfare is a broader term encompassing pig health. When animal welfare is practically evaluated on farms, for example, through an assessment scheme such as the Welfare Quality® protocol, four broad areas are considered. These areas include health, nutrition, environment and behaviour. Thus, besides enjoying good health, pigs should also receive sufficient and appropriate diet, enjoy physical and thermal comfort and have the opportunity to engage in normal non-harmful behaviour directed at the physical environment, their conspecifics and the human caretakers. In combination, all these four areas should result in good animal mental well-being, providing a life in which positive emotional states, such as security, contentment and engagement are promoted while negative states, such as pain, fear, distress, frustration or apathy, are avoided or at least mitigated.

The fact that animal welfare is a more inclusive concept than animal health implies that it is more difficult to agree what is best for pig welfare and how to put it into practice. There is an agreement that advances in pig welfare should be based on evidence, primarily on scientific knowledge. In spite of the progress in applied ethology, neurobiology and comparative psychology, it remains difficult to measure animal behavioural needs and emotional states. Moreover, deciding how to integrate or balance the different aspects of pig welfare is not straightforward. For instance, tail docking causes intense yet relatively short-lived pain in all pigs in the herd (and may even induce more long-term discomfort) yet it reduces the risk of tail-biting outbreaks that may induce severe suffering in a minority of pigs. How should these two aspects of pig welfare be balanced against each other? Free movement of farrowing sows contributes positively to their welfare, through behavioural engagement and positive effects on leg health, yet it may endanger piglet welfare through increased risk of crushing. Again, how should such a trade-off be resolved? These trade-offs in pig welfare are real challenges and the search for answers stimulates research to find innovative solutions. For example, the provision of a stimulating environment and effective monitoring of pig behaviour can reduce tail-biting occurrence in undocked pigs and farrowing pens designed to meet the behavioural needs of both lactating sows and sucking piglets can reduce crushing to levels comparable with crated sows.

At the societal level, the animal welfare discussion is even more complex because it includes not only the matter-of-fact dialogue between professional pig stakeholders (farmers, veterinarians and animal welfare scientists) but also a broader value-related debate with other stakeholders, such as consumers, the food industry and policymakers. With increasing quality of human life, society is gradually becoming more attentive to the well-being of food-producing animals. A genuine dialogue is needed in order to find a common ground and thus to secure the economic, environmental and societal sustainability of pig farming in a dynamically evolving society. On the one hand, broader society needs to have access to accurate information about real pig needs and on the care given to the animals in modern husbandry. On the other hand, pig professionals need to listen to the genuine concerns and expectations society has about farm animals' quality of life and to work on practicable solutions in areas of pig life where the need for progress is most acute.

1.2 A global understanding of animal welfare

REBECCA SOMMERVILLE

Around the world, humans depend on animals for food, transport, entertainment, labour and research. How animals are raised and used for these purposes is influenced by historic traditions combining with modern day influences, which create pressure for change. The resources available, system used, local culture and legislation all combine to influence animal welfare. The welfare status of an individual animal is determined by their health, nutrition, behaviour and environment, which all affect their mental well-being. A global perspective is needed to truly understand animal welfare, as there is no single best location for pig welfare. Pigs reared in an indoor intensive system in a developed country benefit from a veterinarian overseeing their care, temperature controlled barns and welfare legislation. Their ability to express natural behaviour can be restricted, however, if they are not given sufficient space and foraging material. Whereas a pig in a rural smallholding in a less developed country that is free to roam has great behavioural freedom, but their welfare suffers if they become ill and their farmer cannot afford to treat them, or they are malnourished due to a poor-quality diet. In the Global North, indoor intensive systems today provide the majority of pig rearing settings, with a consumer demand for outdoor reared meat at the higher end of the market. In the Global South, traditional smallholding systems remain, which are rapidly being replaced by industrial production in, amongst others, China. Welfare is emerging as a concept in urban areas, creating a demand for more humane systems, as well as for export markets, yet this is restricted by the level of socioeconomic development. A lack of available resources does not necessarily have to be a limiting factor preventing welfare improvement. Training, skills in gentle handling methods and understanding welfare, for example, can facilitate small changes by farmers and stockworkers that can make a big difference to pigs' lives (discussed in detail in Section 4.1). This chapter now discusses animal welfare in different regions around the world and considers how each region's traditions, beliefs, legislation and current consumer trends affect pig welfare.

1.2.1 Europe

HANS A. M. SPOOLDER

European Union (EU) member states have long been the front runners when it comes to animal welfare legislation. The EU itself passed the first directive (on stunning before slaughter) in 1974, and many have followed. Currently there are three pieces of legislation directly addressing pig welfare. They relate to the keeping of pigs (Dir (EU) 58/1998 and Reg (EU) 120/2008), livestock transport (Dir (EU) 1/2005), and stunning and killing of livestock (Dir (EU) 1099/2009). They include several requirements that go beyond what is asked for elsewhere in the world. Examples include a ban on stall housing of pregnant sows after week 4 of pregnancy, the compulsory provision of at least 40 lux of light during 8 hours of the day, and a minimum weaning age of 21 days.

In the last two years, the European Commission has indicated on several occasions that it has no intention of developing new welfare legislation. Although the last EU Strategy for the Protection and Welfare of Animals (2012–2015) still considered the feasibility of introducing a simplified EU legislative framework, a new framework did not materialize. Instead, the Commission is now promoting the guiding principle 'Everyone is Responsible', thus reflecting the obligation and shared interest of all stakeholders to maintain high levels of animal welfare. They are supporting this approach in a number of ways.

First, DG SANTE (the directorate that deals with animal welfare policy) has set up the European Platform on Animal Welfare to 'promote an enhanced dialogue on animal welfare issues that are relevant at EU level among competent authorities, businesses, civil society and scientists' (https://ec.europa.eu/food/animals/welfare/eu-platform-animal-welfare_en). The Platform will focus on better application of EU rules on animal welfare, the development and use of voluntary commitments by businesses, and the promotion of EU animal welfare standards to valorize the market value of EU products. The Platform consists of about 75 members and meets twice per year.

Second, while new legislation is not foreseen, the Commission is pushing for compliance with existing legislation. An important enforcement priority in recent years was the ban on routine docking of pig tails. In the EU tail docking is allowed before day 7 but only in exceptional circumstances. The reality is that more than 95% of EU pigs have their tails cut off. EU member states are now required to produce verifiable action plans to eliminate routine docking, and the progress of these plans is monitored through a programme of inspection visits.

Third, to support farmers, transporters and other stakeholders, DG SANTE organizes activities that develop and disseminate practical advice. An example of this is the 'Animal Transport Guides' project, which produced 'good and better practices' via comprehensive guides, practical factsheets, short videos and a European road show to visit places where transporters meet (www.animaltransportguides.eu). Similarly, support materials were developed to promote welfare at slaughter and the provision of adequate enrichment materials on farm.

Finally, member state policy workers and inspectors are supported through courses included under the 'Better Training for Safer Food' (BTSF) initiative (https://ec.europa.eu/food/safety/btsf_en). In addition, in 2018 the EU Commission designated the first European Reference Centre for Animal Welfare. The centre has a focus on pigs (hence EURCAW-Pigs) and also aims at competent authorities, policy workers and their support bodies. Their website (www.eurcaw.eu) is accessible to all stakeholders and will include scientific and practical knowledge on all areas of EU pig legislation.

1.2.2 North America and Canada

MARINA VON KEYSERLINGK, MARIA CHEN
AND JENNIFER BROWN

In the USA, intensive rearing of pigs is the norm with approximately 75% of sows routinely housed in gestation stalls. Federal US animal welfare legislation includes the Twenty-Eight Hour Law (after 28 hours of travel, livestock must be unloaded into pens with feed and water and rested for at least 5 hours before resuming travel) and the Humane Methods of Slaughter Act, which dictates that livestock must be rendered insensible to pain before slaughter (Office of the Law Revision Counsel, 2002). Although there is a federal Animal Welfare Act, farm animals are excluded from this law (United States Department of Agriculture, 2017). All US states have their own animal cruelty legislation, but most states exempt common agricultural practices. Although interest in animal welfare legislation has increased among the public, the response from animal industry groups has been mixed (von Keyserlingk and Hötzel, 2015). State and local initiatives and bills ('ballot initiatives') initiated by animal protection organizations have gained traction in the USA. For example, the first ballot initiative took place in Florida in 2002 and led to a ban on gestation stalls (effective 2008); as of February 2019, gestation stalls have been banned in 12 US states.

In Canada, industry driven codes of practice form the basis for national standards on the care and handling of farm animals. Species specific codes are created through collaboration between industry representatives, scientists, veterinarians, lay persons and the humane movement. Code development begins with the creation of a scientific report that reviews the relevant scientific research on contentious practices (for example, castration, gestation stalls). Code development follows with input from representatives from all stakeholders, and includes a public consultation period. Each code contains requirements (regulatory or industry-led expectations regarding animal care), as well as recommended best practices. The recently published National Farm Animal Care Council's (NFACC) 2014 Code of Practice for the Care and Handling of Pigs (National Farm Animal Care Council, 2014) has guidelines on general pig care including pain relief to treat post-procedural pain at castration and tail docking, and the provision of environmental enrichment. The document also sets out a ban on the building of new gestation stalls (effective 2014). In an attempt to provide external stakeholders assurance that farmers are adhering to the code guidelines, the Canadian Pork Council has implemented an assurance program that requires all farms to participate. Animal protection law varies across Canada. The federal Criminal Code provides some protection for animals through animal transport regulations, and humane handling and slaughter regulations; abattoirs are inspected by the federal government's Canadian Food Inspection Agency. However, individual provinces also have animal protection laws that include provisions describing a duty of care toward animals; prohibit causing or permitting animal 'distress'; specify exemptions from prosecution; and reference various national and other standards. In most provinces (but not all) on-farm welfare is enforced by the local Society for the Prevention of Cruelty to Animals.

References

National Farm Animal Care Council (2014) Code of practice for the care and handling of pigs. Available at: http://www.nfacc.ca/codes-of-practice/pig-code#preface (accessed 23 January 2019).

Office of the Law Revision Counsel (2002) Chapter 48: Humane methods of livestock slaughter. Available at: http://uscode.house.gov/view.xhtml?hl=false&edition=prelim&path=%2Fprelim%40title7%2Fchapter48&req=granuleid%3AUSC-prelim-title7-chapter48&num=0 (accessed 24 January 2019).

United States Department of Agriculture (2017) Animal welfare act and animal welfare regulations. Available at: https://naldc.nal.usda.gov/download/5969370/PDF (accessed 24 January 2019).

Von Keyserlingk, M.A. and Hötzel, M.J., 2015. The ticking clock: Addressing farm animal welfare in emerging countries. *Journal of Agricultural and Environmental Ethics* 28(1), 179–195.

1.2.3 Asia

CLIVE J. C. PHILLIPS

Asia is a very diverse region with many different approaches to animal welfare and ethics. Part of this derives from different religions, with all the major religions represented. There is a distinct difference between countries adhering to the Abrahamic faiths, Christianity and Islamism, and those adhering to the so-called Eastern religions, Hinduism and Buddhism.

Those conforming to the Abrahamic faiths believe that God placed animals on earth to be used by humans, which gives them a mastery over animals. While welfare may be at a high or low level, humans' absolute right to use animals is not questioned. Those following Eastern religions believe that humans form a continuum with animals, and rebirth as an animal occurs unless, through good deeds, humans can escape the cycle of birth and rebirth and enter heaven. Animals are often gods and a close connection with nature is advocated. Although these religious differences have shaped attitudes to animals across the region, the 20th century saw many turn away from religion and adopt atheistic approaches, particularly in the new-formed Communist countries of China and the Soviet Union, which commonly accepts that animals are used for human benefit.

In addition to these religious influences, attitudes to animal welfare are strongly influenced by culture, hence attitudes are not the same in the Middle East and Indonesia, though both are bastions of Islamism.

In China, the biggest farm animal producer in the world, animal use is accepted by the overwhelming majority of the population, most of whom are atheists, but there is a growing awareness by the urbanized population that animal welfare is important (Figure 1.2). Companion animal ownership is also growing rapidly and influencing attitudes. India, another major user of farm animals, with the biggest dairy cow numbers in the world, has largely retained a strict adherence to Hinduism, which is strongly supportive of both animal welfare and rights. However, in many parts of Asia, poverty still prevails, and human needs tend to be placed before animal needs. Many countries are reducing poverty, particularly in China, and as a result animal welfare is becoming more recognized as a responsibility of the farming community, in particular, as well as of society as a whole.

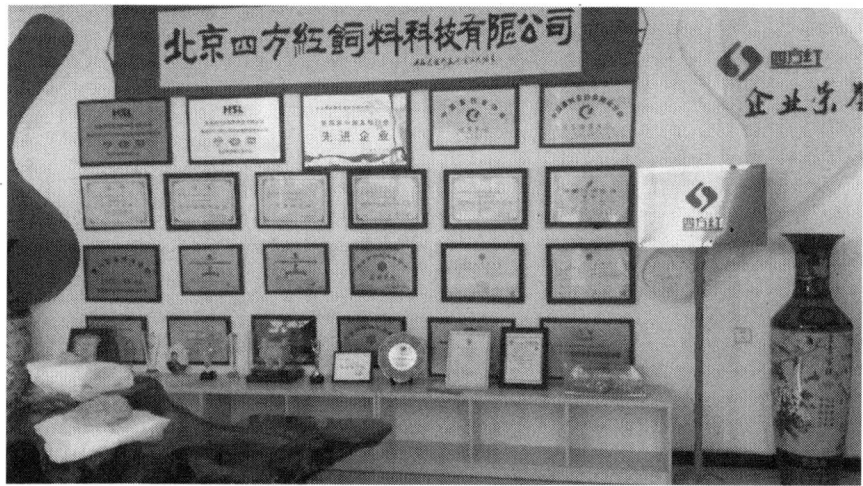

Figure 1.2 Entrance hall with awards at a pig farm near Beijing, China. Good pig management is something to be proud of. Photo: I. Camerlink.

1.2.4 Latin America

MARIA JOSÉ HÖTZEL, RITA ALBERNAZ-GONÇALVES, MARIA CRISTINA YUNES AND DAYANE LEMOS TEIXEIRA

Latin American countries share many characteristics that concern farm animal production and welfare, despite marked cultural, economic and demographic differences across the region. Meat is important in Latin American culture, with many of its countries ranking as high consumers relative to worldwide consumption – though pork still represents a relatively small fraction of all meats consumed. Brazil is a top world producer, consumer and exporter of pork. Mexico, the largest consumer in the region, imports most of its pork. Chile, with a relatively small herd, ranks among the main exporters. Uruguay and Argentina are important players in beef production and trade and meat consumption, but have more modest participation in the pig industry. In most countries, traditional production has been gradually replaced by intensive systems (Figure 1.3), especially regarding monogastrics, even in family farms.

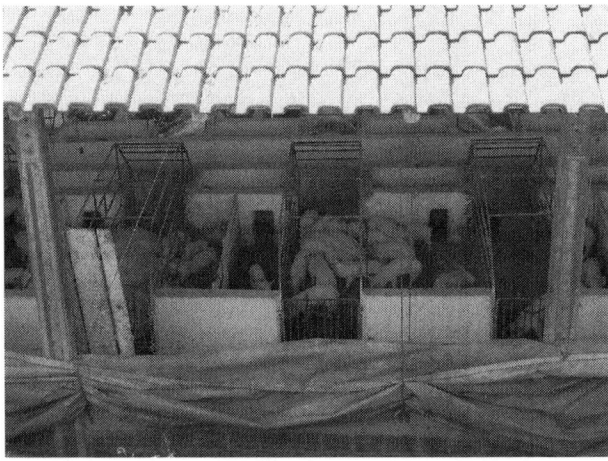

Figure 1.3 Weaner pigs in farrowing pens in Brazil.
Photo: LETA/Universidade Federal de Santa Catarina.

Urbanization has distanced citizens from the reality of animal production. However, when asked for their opinion, consumers show concern about some aspects of the production systems like freedom to move, space, natural behaviours and humane treatment. Given the economic and social relevance of livestock production in Latin American countries, recognizing animal welfare became essential for the sustainability of the animal industries.

Most Latin American countries have laws that protect animals from cruelty, but these laws are not considered effective protection for farm animals. International agreements can be considered the main drivers for change in the region. When the OIE (World Organistion for Animal Health [formerly the Office International des Epizooties]) incorporated farm animal welfare among its missions in the early 2000s, the issue started gaining relevance in science, training, education and regulation; initially this was primarily motivated by trade interests, but soon expanded to the supply chains and the regulatory system of many countries. For instance, in 2003, the first trade agreement to mention animal welfare was the bilateral European Union–Chile agreement. Later on, Chile developed specific rules that protect all food-producing animals in the country during slaughter, transport and industrial production. In Brazil, several decrees and normatives of the Ministry of Agriculture are based on animal welfare principles stated in international agreements to which the country subscribes. Although it does not apply to other production systems, the Brazilian organic production legislation details every step of farm animal production for the main livestock species to ensure animal welfare, which may serve as basis for future regulations. Also, following OIE codes of practice, many Latin American countries have adopted humane slaughter guidelines, though different countries have different levels of enforcement. Finally, following an international trend, national and multinational corporations have announced commitments to change farm animal production practices in a growing number of Latin American countries. The increasing awareness of Latin American citizens, added to these external sources of pressure, are changing livestock production systems in the region.

1.2.5 Australia

CLIVE J. C. PHILLIPS

Australia is a largely urbanized country, with at least 80% of people living in cities, yet it developed only recently, beginning with extensive livestock production on land that was formerly used by aborigines for hunting. This rapid development, over the last 200 years, means that most Australians are concerned about animals' welfare, with their standards based on the companion animals that they now care for. Although most Australians no longer have connections with the land, their recent forebears mostly gained a living from livestock farming. This presents many Australians with a dilemma, they care acutely about the welfare of farm animals, which often have less care given to them than companion animals, yet they recognize that they owe a debt of gratitude to those that farmed livestock. Thus comprehensive animal welfare legislation is necessary in Australia, governed at three levels, federal, state and council.

At a federal level, there is legislation and instruction on the welfare of animals from an international perspective. This includes live export of farm animals and the CITES regulations for endangered species. Australia is also a member of the OIE, which has codes of practice for the welfare of farm animals and dogs that Australia implements at federal and state levels. Australia exports millions of animals to Asia each year to be slaughtered for meat. As implementation of the OIE codes of practice is a matter for individual countries, Australia has been instrumental in encouraging countries that receive live animals exported from Australia to adopt these standards and to manage the animals, particularly at the time of slaughter, in a manner acceptable to the Australian public.

At a state level, there is a legislative framework addressing most concerns about animal welfare, from using animals for sport, for example, horse and dog racing, and organized fighting between animals (the former allowed but controlled, the latter not) to regulations concerning the use of animals in experiments. At a council level, there are local bye-laws governing the management of animals specifically in that council region, for example restrictions on the number of companion animals that can be kept.

1.2.6 Africa

MABEL AWORH-AJUMOBI

Animal welfare in Africa is a new consideration and is usually not considered to be of high priority. Poverty, human starvation, diseases and the low standards of living of the majority of people complicates actions towards better care for animals. Motivating people to adopt good animal welfare practices is a challenge in low-resource settings where poverty, illiteracy, lack of basic healthcare and amenities are perennial problems. In most African countries, there is no enabling legislation to enforce animal welfare standards. Some African countries have made efforts in developing their legislation but enforcing these laws is difficult due to the society's perception of animal welfare. There are thus a lot of challenges to the establishment of good pig welfare in Africa. In some African countries, the presence of animal welfare non-government organizations has made it easier to change human perspectives towards providing animal basic welfare needs.

In addition to traditional rearing of backyard pigs (Figure 1.4), the number of intensive systems are increasing. Intensive pig production systems in most developing economies are usually indoor production systems with an average of 50 or more pigs in total (including sows), use of commercially available feed, and more sophisticated housing with adequate space and pig management is targeted to optimize output. The pig breeds for production are both the better performing exotic and indigenous breeds.

Challenges to good pig welfare in Africa include the following.

- Health problems: poverty has prevented some pig farmers from seeking professional care for their animals.
- Housing problems: some pig farmers are not aware of the basic floor space requirement of pigs, hence both underutilization of space and overcrowding occurs.
- Marketing problems: in Africa, pork is acceptable to some cultures and religions. In countries where the majority is Muslim, pork is usually forbidden. This makes it difficult for pig farmers to break even and remain in business.
- Poor welfare and cruelty to animals are evident at every stage during production, transportation, holdings in the market and slaughter. Transport and handling methods are primitive and crude. Slaughter animals are transported in overcrowded trucks.
- At slaughter, animals are handled roughly and are subjected to unnecessary pain. Animals awaiting slaughter watch other animals being killed. Lack of implementation of existing legislations, as well as religious bias, has led to continued resistance to stunning and inflicting unnecessary pain to the animals.

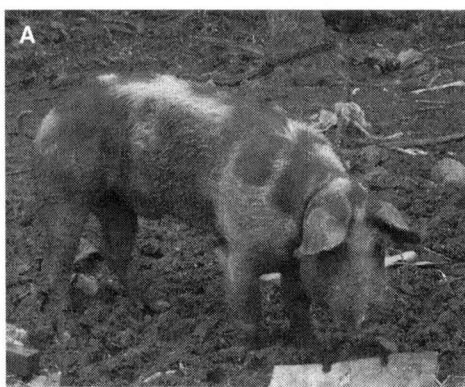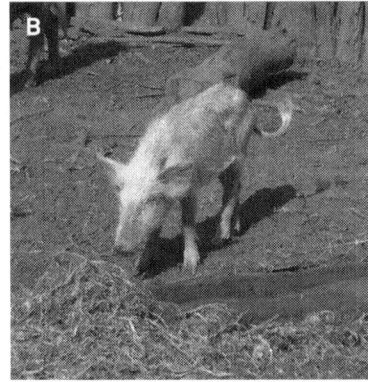

Figure 1.4 A pig in (A) Guadeloupe, Caribbean, tied to a tree and (B) in Guinea Bissau, Africa. Photo: A.A. Almeida.

CHAPTER 2

Making the business case for animal welfare

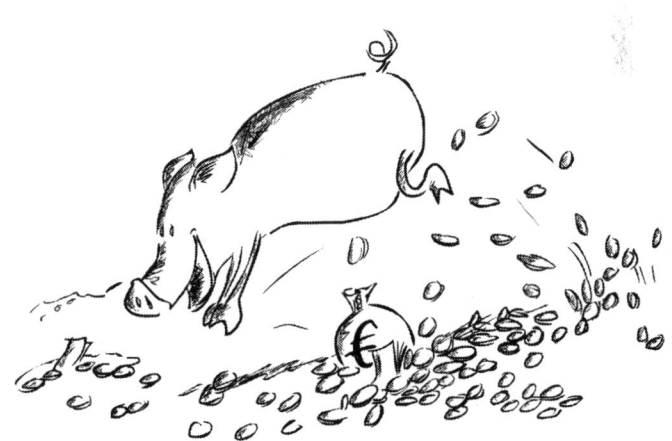

2.1 The profits of improving pig welfare

IRENE CAMERLINK

Researchers often claim that improving animal welfare improves health and productivity. Although, such claims are often based on outcomes under research conditions, similar results come from welfare economics. Calculations using data sets with the average investment and expected productivity result in curves that indicate the optimum balance. For example, the optimum number of pigs per pen to gain maximum profit under improved welfare conditions. Nonetheless, actual numbers remain hard to predict as situations differ across farms and because the sector is changing continuously. Logically, many farmers are sceptical about the returns from improving animal welfare and fear that the improvement in productivity would not return on the investments needed to improve welfare. The aim of this chapter is to give some more insight into the possible returns. Some direct benefits from improving welfare, based on Dawkins (2017), are discussed in this chapter.

2.1.1 Reduced mortality

The highest mortality in pig husbandry is found in the first few days of the piglets' lives. The average mortality is around 12% (in the UK, 2018) but varies widely between farms, showing that improvement is possible. Changes in the farrowing pen or crate design are usually extremely costly and many of the available systems still have their disadvantages. To optimize the costs and benefits it can be more efficient to pay attention to the factors that cause mortality.

A major cause of mortality is piglet crushing by the sow. Keeping calm sows that do not stand up and become restless with every little disturbance reduces the risk of piglets being crushed. Section 2.4 looks at the costs and benefits of conscious gilt rearing and in Chapter 3 more recommendations are given on how to accomplish this.

Neonatal piglets are particularly susceptible to hypothermia, certainly when they do not get immediate access to milk. The provision of a warm and dry piglet nest or creep area and a heat lamp come at a small cost. In hot climates, the temperature should be adjusted to respect the thermal comfort zone of piglets as well as sows.

Reducing mortality by reducing the occurrence of tail biting is another way in which improving animal welfare translates into improved profitability. In Section 2.3 an analysis is given of the costs of tail biting.

2.1.2 Improved health

Sick animals will require more medication and will have a reduced feed efficiency. Improving health directly contributes to welfare but the converse is also true. Long-term stress may suppress immune responses. Increasing welfare through reducing stress may therefore improve disease resistance in pigs. Chapter 4 looks at possible ways to reduce stress. Good welfare will also reduce the risk of zoonoses and animal-born infections. The benefits of good welfare can be seen in reduced veterinary costs and reduced medication. The latter will also contribute to avoiding or limiting the development of antibiotics resistance. This is also an important consideration for your own health as unfortunately not only pigs but also many pig farmers test positive on the presence of MRSA (methicillin-resistant staphylococcus aureus).

2.1.3 Improved product quality

For pigs the transition from farm to the slaughter plant is per definition stressful as it includes encounters with unfamiliar pigs (fighting), feed/water restriction, transport and potentially rough handling. The accumulated stress and injuries can cause condemnation and devaluing of the carcass (see also Section 3.1.6 on skin lesion at slaughter). An extreme case of this was seen in pigs with the halothane gene. These pigs showed a reduced meat quality (pale and high drip loss) and especially so when they were stressed.

Good results are obtained with specialized on-farm slaughter or company-owned slaughter plants near to the production site. Unfortunately, in many cases the distance to the slaughter plant and the way the pigs are handled on the truck and lairage is often outside the farmer's influence. Small improvements that are within the farmer's influence include: (1) avoiding stress pre-transport by not regrouping pigs beforehand; (2) reducing fearfulness towards humans (Section 4.1); and (3) calm handling when moving pigs onto the truck.

2.1.4 Increased job satisfaction

Seeing healthy and happy animals contributes to increased job satisfaction. Although this does not often translate into financial benefits in the short term, this does become relevant in the long term for companies with staff. Companies may struggle to find good staff and often face a high employee turnover. Increasing employee job satisfaction may result in lower turnover, which reduces the costs of recruiting and training new staff.

2.1.5 Commanding higher prices from consumers

Consumers appreciate better quality products and regard better welfare standards as one aspect that improves product quality. Consistently across studies and countries, consumers' actual willingness to pay is much lower than what they state when asked about this: often less than £1.50/kg (~€2) higher for meat products from a better welfare origin compared to a standard product. Small-scale rural farms as well as large-scale companies can improve revenues by selling pork directly to their customers (and avoid retail taking the main profits). Marketing of niche products of high quality, such as the meat from slow growing pig breeds (Figure 2.1), can command a much higher price even through retail when good branding is applied. The cost of raising such pigs is, however, also higher.

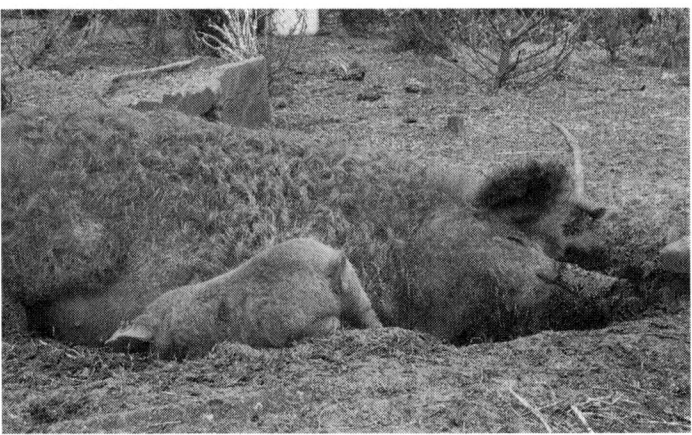

Fig 2.1 The slow growing Mangalitsa pig has a very good meat quality and great appeal to local citizens, making it ideal for special branding and sales of pork directly from farm to customers. Photo: Moderne Oerboerderij Spek.

Reference

Dawkins, M.S. (2017) Animal welfare and efficient farming: is conflict inevitable? *Animal Production Science* 57(2), 201–208. Available at: http://www.publish.csiro.au/AN/AN15383 (accessed 6 July 2019).

2.2 Animal welfare, society and economics

JOHN STRAK

As far as farmers are concerned any official regulation or legal standard that is applied to their production system is almost certainly going to increase their costs. In practice, it is hard to think of a new government regulation that reduces costs and hence the general cry that we hear from farmers (and businesses) is, 'get rid of the red tape!'. Rules governing animal welfare have often been the focus of such protest, although, it is fair to point out that many government rules have the same effect on costs as welfare ones. Laws on: food safety; payment and treatment of employees; the self-employed; health and safety in the workplace; and on the environment (pollution, recycling, waste disposal and so on) essentially all tend to increase production costs. The purpose of this section is to consider why these rules tend to get more numerous and far reaching over time, and how and when they should be considered a threat to a farmer's business, and why they are here to stay.

First of all, let us deal with the basic question, why do governments (of all political persuasions) introduce new laws? A little reflection provides an obvious answer to this – because the voters want them. And even in authoritative regimes where the voters may not have a loud voice, we see government officials and politicians introducing laws that govern how businesses and consumers go about their daily lives. We do not need to be well read historians to recognize that, over time, the voters reflect different concerns in society and, crucially, that their per capita incomes and purchasing power rise. Over centuries a modern developed economy will build numerous laws and regulations that affect the costs of business.

Some British examples from the last 200 years are instructive: the Adulteration of Food and Drink Act 1860 made it an offence to knowingly sell food that endangers health or is adulterated in any way (this Act was followed by several others in the 1870s); the Factory Act 1878 prohibited work before the age of 10 and applied to all trades; in 1956 the Clean Air Act was introduced; and in 1974 the Health and Safety at Work Act went on the statute. All of these laws increased the costs of doing business. Less obviously cost-increasing but, nevertheless, affecting the behaviour of business and consumers other examples are: the Abolition of Slavery Act 1833, and the Cruelty to Animals Act 1835, which introduced a ban on bear baiting. Economic development also leads to increased lobbying of government. In 1840 Queen Victoria gave permission to add the royal R to the Society for the Prevention of Cruelty to Animals – a group that had been formed in a London coffee shop in 1824. The RSPCA has thus been around for almost 200 years and is a symbol of British society's interest in the welfare of animals.

While not all of these laws and regulations may have been brought in by a groundswell of popular support and, indeed, some elements of them may still not be popular, it is unthinkable for modern society to repeal these laws. Why? Because a modern society recognizes that the outcomes that these regulations deliver are desirable. Society also implicitly recognizes that it is prepared to pay for (and generally can afford) these outcomes. We see this in developed economies across Europe and North America, and we also see the adoption of these regulations in emerging and developing economies (usually at the pace that a particular economy can afford). Global consumers have, over time, expressed their views about the safety of their food and how they want to see animals treated, and in some countries legislators have reacted by bringing in new laws. Some changes to the law may have been instigated by pressure groups (like animal protection groups) and those lobby groups may have acted in advance of majority consumer opinion. But the fact that there has been no clamour from the general population to revoke laws introduced as a result of the pressure from small groups of voters speaks volumes. Indeed, societies everywhere are showing little sign of wanting to go back to the former ways of farming.

This observation brings us to the second area of debate – who pays for all this? Economics can offer some guidance on the impact of government regulations. A cost-increasing regulation will, in the long run, increase the price of a product and, unless technology reduces costs in some other part of the cost function, that means higher prices for consumers. Consumers have a choice – to pay all of this extra cost by continuing to purchase the same amount of the product at the new higher price, or (more likely) to reduce their demand as prices rise and thus share the impact of the higher price between consumers and producers. In other words, consumers buy a smaller amount at a higher price and producers sell fewer units. Producers also have the choice of passing on part or all of the extra cost – thus keeping prices down and maintaining sales – but would have to counter this by reducing costs elsewhere through improved efficiency.

If we take animal welfare as the example, a new welfare regulation for pigs that increases costs for pig farmers means that the price of pork should rise to reflect this. If it does and if consumers continue to buy the same amount of pork the impact on farmers will be zero – all of the extra costs are borne by consumers. But, of course, it is not that simple in practice because consumers can substitute, and, sometimes, government laws (inadvertently) encourage such substitution.

Substitution between products is seen in all aspects of production and consumption and the food sector offers daily examples of such behaviour – as a trip to any supermarket will confirm. Consumers can substitute between different proteins (meat, fish, eggs, vegetable protein) and between proteins, carbohydrates and fats. They can substitute between classes of protein (pork, beef, chicken) and between a long list of fruits, vegetables, grains and oilseeds. And, significantly, the main driver of substitution for most consumers is price. In other words, it is likely that any increase in the price of pork because of new animal welfare rules will lead to some reduced demand for pig farmers as consumers switch to beef, chicken and other protein sources (assuming no price or quality changes in these alternatives). It gets worse. In an open economy where there is international trade in goods there will be imports of foreign pork to the domestic market. This may be restricted by transport costs for fresh and chilled products but any frozen or semi-processed products (ham, bacon, cooked meats) will be direct substitutes for similar domestic products. And if those foreign suppliers do not have to meet the same welfare standards as domestic producers, then that suggests another source of substitutes for domestic consumers: Danish or Dutch bacon for British bacon for example. Yes, of course, those consumers are the same ones that earlier said that they wanted the new laws brought in by government and this paradoxical behaviour is a threat to pig farmers. The inapplicability of domestic animal welfare laws to international trade and the paradox of consumer behaviour need to be recognized by farmers in their business planning.

The World Trade Organization (WTO) and the EU's Single Market do not recognize animal welfare as a legitimate reason for a country to restrict or ban imports (the debate is ongoing). The EU insists on certain EU-approved minimum standards in animal welfare, but if a country has domestic legislation that imposes a higher standard this cannot be used to restrict trade from other member states. For example, the ban on sow stalls in the UK in 1999 occurred long before a similar ban was introduced in the rest of the EU in 2013. The result was an increase in farmers' costs and a growth in imports from the rest of the EU, as supermarkets (consumers) sought to avoid any increase in the costs of pork by switching to other sources of meat protein. The size of the UK pig herd, the number of pig farmers and investment fell sharply in the early part of the 21st century and these measures of pig industry health have not recovered.

The paradox identified above is key to pig farmers' profitability and needs to be recognized. There is plenty of evidence that the paradox exists and it may depress farmers to know that consumers vote for one thing in the ballot box (for higher animal welfare) and vote with their wallets in the supermarket aisle (for the cheapest piece of pork). This is true in general but a deeper look at consumer motivations for a purchase decision recognizes that many other factors are becoming more important to consumer demand in a modern society. Consumers, of course, want convenience and healthy foods but they also want provenance, taste and flavour, Fairtrade and 'climate change friendly' products. These other drivers are often highly correlated with ethical, high animal welfare productions systems. In short, farmers might do better to sell their products by overtly offering these characteristics rather than just being labelled as, 'welfare friendly'. Such a strategy may reduce the impact of the paradox observed in the past for high welfare animal production and also reduce the opportunities for substitution by foreign suppliers.

Consumer purchasing behaviour is becoming more complex as global society develops and recognizes new attributes, which is observed in the way that demand for (food) products is expressed. Farmers will need to respond to this on the farm and at the point of sale by becoming equally complex. The push for improved animal welfare is part of a more complex and sophisticated consumer demand function, and farm production systems operated by progressive farmers need to respond to this. There is no going back to the 'good old days'.

2.3 The costs of tail damage

RICK B. D'EATH

Tail biting is an unpredictable and costly problem. On-farm costs include pigs that die or are euthanized, and veterinary treatments for tail injuries. There are costs of providing hospital pens for injured pigs and staff costs for monitoring, moving and treating bitten pigs. Other than removing bitten or biting pigs, there are costs to adding additional enrichment materials, such as straw or silage in racks, ropes or shredded paper, to the pen to occupy pigs and prevent further biting. At slaughter, there is a considerable cost for entire or partial carcass condemnations as a result of tail biting. We recently estimated these costs to average at €19 per tail biting victim pig (D'Eath et al., 2016; Figure 2.2).

Tail docking is not a complete solution, but it is effective at reducing the damage associated with tail biting, and is relatively cheap to carry out (equipment is inexpensive, cost is mainly in staff time). As such it is widely used in the industry.

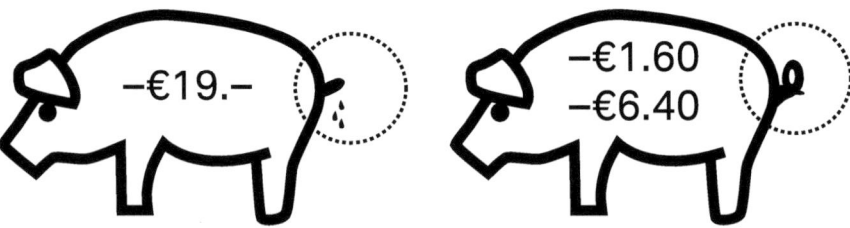

Figure 2.2 Costs of having a tail bitten victim and of keeping pigs with long tails. Illustration: L. van der Zande.

However, tail docking raises ethical concerns for consumers and governments. It is only allowed as a last resort in the EU. The provision of more space and enrichment materials, such as straw, to reduce the risk of tail biting to acceptable levels without docking can increase costs. By comparing Finnish (undocked) and Danish (docked) production conditions, we calculated increased production costs for undocked pigs to be in the region of €1.60 to €6.40 per pig (based on 109 kg at slaughter and 82 kg yield).

To offset these costs, farmers need to get a premium price for the pig. Fortunately, raising pigs with intact tails can increase the sale price of the finished pig as part of farm assurance schemes with consumer labelling on pork products in various countries. These schemes have a number of requirements for membership other than stopping tail docking.

In the UK, the RSPCA Assured scheme does not allow tail docking, except as a last resort. Pig producers must apply for permission to dock, and can be required for up to 1 year to try other steps and cease docking. The price premium is around £0.07–£0.10 (€0.08–€0.11) per kg or £5.74–£8.20 (€6.60–€9.43) per finished pig. In the Netherlands, the Beter Leven scheme does not allow tail docking at all, and offers 3 'starred' levels of accreditation. Denmark's similar 3 level Bedre Dyrevelfaerd (Better Animal Welfare) also bans tail docking. There is a price premium of DKK 1.4 per kg (2 hearts level = Antonius production, €0.18 per kg). Germany's Initiative Tierwohl offers several options through which farmers can gain extra payments for changes that benefit animal welfare. Stopping docking is not on the list, however. Providing 10, 20 or 40% more than the minimum space allowance provides a premium of €0.80, 1.20 or 2.40 per pig, and permanent access to roughage, such as straw or hay €0.40, or additional organic materials €0.30. Taking some or all of these steps would reduce the need for tail docking. These schemes make it possible to offset the increased production costs associated with improving pig welfare through better environments which reduce tail biting risk, reducing the need to tail dock.

Reference

D'Eath, R.B., Niemi, J.K., Ahmadi, B.V., Rutherford, K.M.D., Ison, S.H., Turner, S.P., Anker, H.T., Jensen, T., Busch, M.E., Jensen, K.K. and Lawrence, A.B. (2016) Why are most EU pigs tail docked? Economic and ethical analysis of four pig housing and management scenarios in the light of EU legislation and animal welfare outcomes. *Animal* 10(4), 687–699.

2.4 Cost–benefit analysis: gilt rearing

IRENE CAMERLINK

Good sows are the basis of a good pig herd. In order to keep good sows, it is important to invest time into the current sows' health and welfare, but also to consciously select the future generations of gilt. Here a calculation is given for how this can pay off.

2.4.1 The influence of human handling

Sows are easily distressed by human interference. Their nervousness and defensiveness partly depends on the breed or genetic line, but is largely determined by them being used to humans or not. Often the only association sows have with humans is negative (rough handling, injections, handling piglets). This makes them call the alarm whenever a human enters the farrowing house. To change this, the sows need to get a neutral or positive association to humans. To get calm sows in the farrowing house it is important to start at the gilt rearing. Calm and positive human–animal contact does not need to take much time. Positive effects on behaviour can be seen by scratching the sow behind the ears for 15 seconds upon inspection (see also Section 4.1). Calm sows will stand up less frequently and this reduces the risk of crushing. They will also vocalize less, and therefore cause fewer disturbances to neighbouring sows including those nursing.

2.4.2 Selecting for calm behaviour

Behavioural traits are moderately heritable. That means that it is possible to reduce aggression and increase calm behaviour on farm by genetically selecting against it. To do so it is best to start from the sow population by giving each sow at the day of piglet handling a score of 1–3 for their response when catching the piglets for processing. An example of a simple scoring system could be 1: calm; 2: responding but not aggressive; 3: aggressive towards humans. Note the score on the sow card for future reference or in a record where sow performance is evaluated. It is best not to keep sows that show score 3. Defensive sows can be very good mothers by being attentive to the piglets, but that should not be the only criteria for keeping them. Although they may raise good piglets, the effect of their defensive behaviour may cost more in the long term. The nervous defensive behaviour of this sow may indirectly result in loss of piglets from other sows due to crushing and it is therefore not beneficial per se to keep such sows. Further down the line the sow's behaviour may also result in more aggression or nervousness in the growing pigs, which can increase the costs of this behaviour.

2.4.3 Strategy to gain good sows

To be able to select for good replacement gilts there needs to be choice. Only inseminating the minimum number of sows with dam line semen may make it impossible to select for good replacement gilts within the number of female piglets born. Inseminating more sows with dam line semen will give leaner, slower growing pigs for slaughter but this will be compensated by having better sows in future. Select female dam line piglets at weaning for teat number, good leg strength and good body condition. Skin lesions on the front part of the body indicate active involvement in fights and when having the choice it is best not to select piglets with skin lesions on the front of the body.

2.4.4 The cost–benefit of investing in good sows

Let us suppose that a good sow gives on average one piglet more per year than a bad sow. This seems a realistic number as stressed or less careful sows easily lose a piglet due to crushing, savaging or poor milk production. Selecting on strong legs will also increase the longevity of the sow. This is not calculated here due to lack of information on economic consequences of lameness. However, a reduction in lameness will reduce costs of treatment and culling, and will reduce the required percentage of replacement gilts. The following calculation is based on average numbers of pig production in UK. Prices will of course fluctuate and depend on overall performance. In the example of a 100 sow herd, twice the number of sows is inseminated with dam line semen in order to have the possibility of selecting replacement gilts on preferred characteristics. This prevents the need to replace sows with lower quality gilts due to lack of choice, or being forced to keep sows that would better be replaced. The net benefit of this choice would be £313.80 per 100 sows. The main take home message is therefore to make decisions that bring long-term benefits, those that improve the pig herd as a whole.

Table 2.1 Input variables.

Number of sows on farm	100
Replacement gilts needed (%)	30
Pigs weaned per litter by F1 sows (50% of litter ♀)	10 (5 ♀)
Difference in growth to slaughter between dam line (Landrace) and crossbred (Yorkshire type)[a]	+20 days
Average cost price/pig/day (£115/pig[b] for 150 days to market[c])	£0.77
Estimated net margin in UK /head (2017)[d]	£12

Notes: [a]Bell, J. M. (1964) A study of rates of growth of Yorkshire, Lacombe, Landrace, and crossbred pigs from birth to 200 lb. *Canadian Journal of Animal Science* 44(3), 315–319; [b]https://www.pork.org/facts/stats/costs-and-prices/ or 1.26 gbp/kg dead weight (ADHB Pork; https://pork.ahdb.org.uk/media/274535/2016-pig-cost-of-production-in-selected-countries.pdf); [c]http://www.thepigsite.com/stockstds/3/pig-farm-targets/; [d]https://pork.ahdb.org.uk/media/274535/2016-pig-cost-of-production-in-selected-countries.pdf.

Table 2.2 Costs and benefits of careful selection of gilts.

	Standard selection		Careful selection	
	Cost	Benefit	Cost	Benefit
Inseminate with dam line semen	6 sows		12 sows	
Dam line pigs not used for replacement[a]	30 pigs		90 pigs	
Loss due to slower growth of dam line pigs[b]	−£23.10		−£69.30	
Pigs weaned / gilt		0		+1
Total piglets from gilts[c]		300		330
Profit from piglets of gilts		£3,600		£3,960
Net benefit[d]		£3,576		£3,890

Notes: [a]n sows × n weaned pigs − n selected gilts; [b]n slower growing pigs × 0.77; [c]% replacement gilts × n piglets weaned; [d]benefit − costs.

2.5 Economic evaluation of farrowing systems

YOLANDE SEDDON

The farrowing crate is the most widely used indoor system for housing sows during parturition and lactation. The restriction of the sow is favoured for ease of management, worker safety and reduction of the risk of piglet crushing. Yet, because the farrowing crate interferes with the expression of maternal behaviours and limits the transfer of information between the sow and her piglets, the use of the farrowing crate continues to raise welfare concerns, and is unfavourably viewed by the consumer.

Research efforts within the last 10–15 years have focused on developing commercially viable systems that can deliver for higher welfare, performance, worker safety and efficiency of management. The result is an explosion of system variations that offer something a little different. This section will explore how the cost of producing an 8 kg piglet varies in these systems.

2.5.1 Alternative indoor farrowing system costs

Different farrowing pen systems are described in detail in Section 4.6.2 and on www.freefarrowing.org and here only the information regarding the cost calculation is provided. Group lactation systems will not be covered here.

Economic concerns over the adoption of alternative farrowing systems include not only the initial investment costs, but the longer-term running costs, considering the performance achievable in such systems. To support informed decision making, a spreadsheet-based financial model was developed by researchers at Newcastle University, UK, to estimate the cost of producing a weaner pig in several, commercially viable, alternative farrowing systems, when compared to existing farrowing crate systems. The methods and specifications of the model are described by Seddon et al. (2013). Producers can input their own productivity data into this model to explore the cost of production in various system combinations. This model is available for use on the free farrowing website: www.freefarrowing.org.

In brief, capital building costs of systems were obtained from farm building companies, with costs amortized (paid in instalments) based on an interest rate of 8% over the building lifetime, providing an annualized charge. Annual repair costs were estimated from farm building survey data and used to calculate a repair factor, as a percentage of the capital building value and applied to the capital costs determined. Standard unit prices for feedstuffs, labour and machinery were calculated from a farm business costings guide, and energy use from farm surveys and energy monitoring at Newcastle University pig unit (UK). Labour inputs for the PigSAFE system versus crates collated during the PigSAFE research project (UK) suggested labour was similar between the two systems. Given the lack of labour data on alternative farrowing systems in literature, labour inputs were kept the same across systems (Seddon et al., 2013). At the time of development, this model produces figures similar to the cost of production reported for commercial farms as reported in the UK, BPEX (now AHDB Pork) Pig Yearbook (BPEX, 2010).

The standard farrowing crate, and four alternative indoor farrowing systems costed in the model are shown in Table 2.3. Each differ in the quantity of space available for the sow and her litter, the ability to restrain the sow, and the level of protection awarded to the producer.

Table 2.3 Specification and building costs of different farrowing systems.

Variable	Crate	360° Freedom Farrower	Swing-side crate	Danish[c]	PigSAFE[c]
Area (m²)	4.3	4.3	5.7	6	8.9
Crating	Always	Temp.[d]	Temp.	No	Feeder[e]
Flooring[a]	FS	FS	FS	PS	PS
Bedding[b]	N	N	N	MS	MS
Cost[f]	3170	3670	3771	3804	4388
Lifetime (years)	20	20	20	20	20
Cost diff.[g]	0	500	601	634	1218
% diff.[h]	0	16	19	20	38

Notes: [a]FS = fully slatted, PS = part slatted; [b]MS = minimal straw provision; [c]specified with one access passageway, as opposed to two; [d]temporary; [e]lockable feeder; [f]capital cost in £ per place; [g]compared to crate (£ per place); [h]change in capital cost from crate (%).

The 360˚ Freedom Farrower™ (Dalgety Farm systems, UK) utilizes the same building space area for the sow and litter as a farrowing crate (4.3 m²), but has a 16% greater capital cost due to a more expensive crate, with a sophisticated hinge mechanism allowing it to open, width-wise. Swing-side crates typically have a slightly larger space allowance for sow and litter, and the area of 5.7 m² per sow was costed from the average of two swing crates on the market. The simple swing-crate design is not much more than a standard farrowing crate, but the increased space increases the capital cost per place by 19%. By comparison, cost of constructing a Danish pen system (JLF10, Jyden Bur Staldinventar, Denmark) is only 1% greater than the swing crate, or 20% greater than the farrowing crate. The PigSAFE pen has the greatest capital cost, being 38% higher than the cost of a crate, and largely due to a total increased building space, and design features such as the lockable feeder. In commercial adoption of the PigSAFE system, a number of producers have chosen to modify the design, removing the use of the feeding stall for example. As such, the Danish system, without such a feeder, illustrates a comparable design in commercial adoption. For adoption of designed pens, the design and size of the nest site (the solid floored area) is very important. Nest design and size has been well researched, and should not be altered. Modification of the nest design can change the lying behaviour of the sow, which can lead to increased piglet mortality.

Assuming a sow herd size of 545 sows, with an average live-born litter-size of 11.59 piglets, and 2.25 litters/sow/year, the cost of producing an 8 kg piglet in five indoor farrowing system designs, at three different levels of pre-weaning live-born mortality, when assuming a common gestation sow system (straw yard, with a scrap through passageway and dump feeding system) is given in Table 2.4.

Assuming a 12% pre-weaning live-born mortality, the cost of producing a piglet in the PigSAFE system is 3.5% greater than in a standard crate. With a smaller building footprint, producing a piglet in a temporary crating system, is only 1.6% greater than the cost in a crate. However,

Table 2.4 Cost of production (total gestation and farrowing costs, £), and percentage difference to the crate, per sow and per 8 kg piglet produced, at different levels of pre-weaning live-born mortality in five different indoor farrowing systems.

Live born mortality		Crate	360° Freedom Farrower	Swing-side crate	Danish	PigSAFE
	Sow	788.44	800.59	801.58	801.48	815.80
12%	8 kg pig	34.57	35.10	35.14	35.14	35.77
10%	8 kg pig	33.80	34.32	34.36	34.35	34.97
15%	8 kg pig	35.79	36.34	36.39	36.38	37.03
% difference		0	1.5%	1.7%	1.6%	3.5%

the Danish pen has also only 1.6% greater costs than a traditional crate system. Costs are largely due to the increased building costs. The model assumes equal sow feed intake across systems, however, there are anecdotal reports that sow feed intake may increase in loose systems, which in turn could support improved lactation output.

2.5.2 Reducing costs

Increased piglet mortality is one of the greatest concerns of having a sow farrow loose. A temporary increase in mortality is not unexpected as staff and sows adjust to the new system. If live-born mortality were to increase to 15%, the cost of producing a piglet rises markedly, with a 7% increase for the PigSAFE system, and around 5% increase for the 360° Freedom Farrower, swing-side crate and Danish pen. Research into the commercial adoption of indoor loose farrowing systems has identified that temporary restraint of the sow for up to 4 days post-farrowing can support a reduction in pre-weaning live-born mortality (Hales et al., 2015). Temporary crating designs, the 360° Freedom Farrower and the swing-side crate offer the ability to confine the sow in the days around farrowing. The free farrowing pens do not enable temporary restriction of the sow, and therefore, efforts to rapidly achieve optimal management are important to manage the cost of production. Danish researchers have developed the SWAP pen (Sow Welfare and Piglet Protection), a modification of the Danish free farrowing pen, in which the front of the creep swings round to restrict the sow for the first few days after farrowing, providing a flexible option to help reduce crushing.

When the crate is open, the most important aspects of the design are the total available space for the sow and piglets, pen features that support sow lying behaviour (such as sloped walls) and features that reduce piglet crushing. Such features may be a better investment than systems that offer temporary crating without these features. However, currently, there remains insufficient data of mortality in temporary crating systems to evaluate this.

While production data can vary widely per farm, commercial trials of the designed pens have found live-born mortality can be comparable, and in some instances, better, than that of crates. Commercial trials of the PigSAFE pen show that once stockpeople are comfortable with the system, a pre-weaning, live-born mortality of 10% is achievable, exceeding performance of the farrowing crate. Should pre-weaning mortality be reduced to 10%, the cost of producing a piglet in a free farrowing pen reduces to 1.2% greater (PigSAFE), or –0.6% lower (Danish), than the cost of producing a piglet in a standard farrowing crate at 12% live-born mortality.

Research trials of alternative farrowing system designs have identified that when the sow is loose during farrowing and lactation, a higher weaning weight of typically 0.3 kg/piglet is achieved. An economic analysis identified that this improvement in weaning weights would reduce the cost of production by 0.9% in the PigSAFE system compared to a standard farrowing crate, as measured by cost of production in pence per kilogram of carcass weight produced (Cain et al., 2013).

2.5.3 Business goals

Prior to investment into an alternative farrowing system, you should consider longer-term welfare goals alongside the productivity goals of your operation. Regarding pig welfare goals, the major criticism of the farrowing crate is restriction of the sow around farrowing. Therefore, a system in which the sow can nest build and farrow loose addresses this. In a loose system, the sow's mothering abilities should be utilized to support reductions in mortality. Substrate provided prior to farrowing allows the sow to fully express this maternal care behaviour, and is associated with lower numbers of stillborn, starved and crushed piglets (Ocepek and Andersen, 2018).

The space per sow differs in each of the pen designs, and it is space that brings the main cost. However, if you aim to increase litter size, adopting a system with a larger space for sow and litter may be more beneficial.

2.5.4 Conclusion

Assuming a comparable level of mortality, alternative farrowing system designs will increase the cost of production in comparison to the standard farrowing crate, and markedly so if piglet mortality increases. However, when optimizing management, data from the commercial adoption of some pen designs indicates mortality performance at the level of crates is achievable with higher piglet wean weights.

References

BPEX (British Pig Executive) (2010) *Pig Yearbook 2010*, Kenilworth, BPEX.

Cain, P.J., Guy, J.G., Seddon, Y., Baxter, E.M. and Edwards, S.E. (2013) Estimating the economic impact of the adoption of novel non-crate sow farrowing systems in the UK. *International Journal of Agricultural Management* 2(2), 113–118.

Hales, J., Moustsen, V.A., Devreese, A.M., Nielsen, M.B.F. and Hansen, C.F. (2015) Comparable farrowing progress in confined and loose housed hyperprolific sows. *Livestock Science* 171, 64–72.

Ocepek, M. and Andersen, I.L. (2018) Sow communication with piglets while being active is a good predictor of maternal skills, piglet survival and litter quality in three different breeds of domestic pigs (*Sus scrofa domesticus*). *PloS one* 13(11), p.e0206128.

Seddon, Y.M., Cain, P.J., Guy, J.H. and Edwards, S.A. (2013) Development of a spreadsheet based financial model for pig producers considering high welfare farrowing systems. *Livestock Science* 157(1), 317–321.

2.6 Make your own cost–benefit analysis

RACHEL S. E. PEDEN

Cost–benefit analysis is a popular tool used for weighing up benefits and the associated costs of a project, in order to decide whether or not to go ahead. The previous sections described examples of how cost–benefit analysis can be applied to the animal welfare issues of tail biting (Section 2.3) and gilt rearing (Section 2.4) on the farm. In this section, we provide step-by-step instructions, and describe the important things that you should take into consideration, when doing your own cost–benefit analysis. Specifically, you will obtain a preliminary estimate of the monetary consequences of implementing a new animal welfare measure. The monetary consequences of this measure can then be compared to alternative measures, in order to decide on the most appropriate route to take on your farm. This guide will, therefore, help you answer questions such as the following.

- Do the benefits of this animal welfare measure exceed its costs?
- Of alternative animal welfare measures, which one achieves the greatest benefit when compared to cost?

Go through the following steps.

1. Define a time frame. The time frame defines how far into the future you will measure costs and benefits, for example, over the following 1 month, 6 months, 1 year, 2 years or 5 years.

2. Make a list of all foreseeable costs over your time frame as best you can based on the information available. Remember, that there will be initial investments costs but also ongoing costs.

3. Make a list of all foreseeable benefits over your time frame as best you can based on the information available. See Tip 1 below.

4. Assign a monetary value to each cost over your time frame.

5. Assign a monetary value to each benefit over your time frame. See Tips 2–4 below.

6. Subtract the costs from the benefits. Do the benefits of this animal welfare measure outweigh the costs? See Tip 5 below.

7. Compare to alternatives. Are there any alternative measures you could make? Repeat steps 1–6 for all alternative measures. Which one has the greatest benefits in comparison to costs?

8. Compare the results to doing nothing. Are you at a disadvantage if you keep your current practice, compared to if you implement a new measure?

5 TIPS

1. Some costs and benefits may be unanticipated. Can you envisage any hidden costs or benefits? See Table 2.5 for some ideas.

2. Depending on your chosen time frame, there are things to take into consideration, for example, for longer time frames (5 years) there will be more fluctuation in pig prices, there may also be opportunities for subsidies, whereas for shorter time frames (1 month) the current pig prices need to be considered and not an average.

3. Some costs and benefits may not have an obvious monetary value, but try to think about the bigger picture, for example, improved job satisfaction can lead to improved staff retention, and this saves money on training new staff.

4. When estimating your monetary values, seek advice from other farmers who have used the measure, and veterinarians and researchers.

5. Uncertainty is inherent. In order to go ahead with a new animal welfare measure on your farm, the benefits should exceed the costs (it should more than break even).

Table 2.5 Potential costs and benefits of animal welfare measures.

Costs	Benefits
Start-up costs:	Improved feed efficiency
Investment in new materials	Improved growth rate
Farm restructuring	Improved job satisfaction (staff retention)
Staff training	Greater number of weaned pigs
Ongoing costs:	Easier animal handling
Increased staff workload	Reduced mortality
Maintenance/cleaning of equipment	Reduced labour requirements
Replenishment of materials	Reduced veterinary costs

Animal welfare measure:			
Timeframe: 1 month / 6 months / 1 year / 2 years / 5 years			
Costs	Monetary estimate (£,€)	Benefits	Monetary estimate (£,€)
1.		1.	
2.		2.	
3.		3.	
4.		4.	
5.		5.	
Total costs:		**Total benefits:**	
Total benefits − total costs =			

CHAPTER 3

Assessing animal welfare

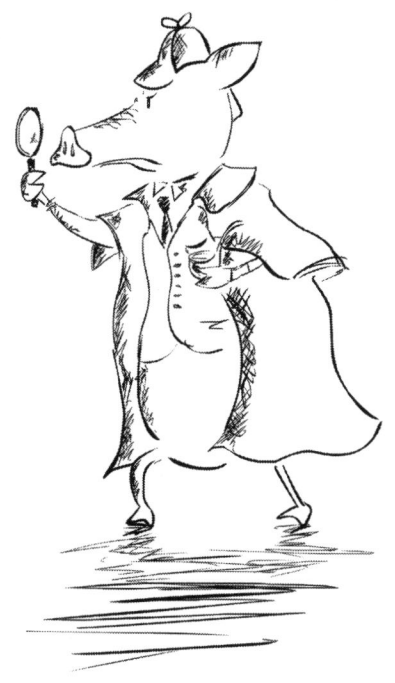

3.1 Iceberg indicators

Animal welfare cannot be reflected in one single measure. That is why welfare assessment protocols are often long. Welfare is instead reflected in a multitude of outcomes, including external conditions, such as housing, and animal-based outcomes, such as health and behaviour. There are, however, several measures that show up with various animal welfare problems. They therefore reflect not just one welfare aspect but reveal that there may be a greater and diverse problem underneath. These measures show the 'tip of the iceberg' of animal welfare and are therefore called *iceberg indicators* (Figure 3.1). In this chapter experts describe several iceberg indicators and how you can use them for improving welfare.

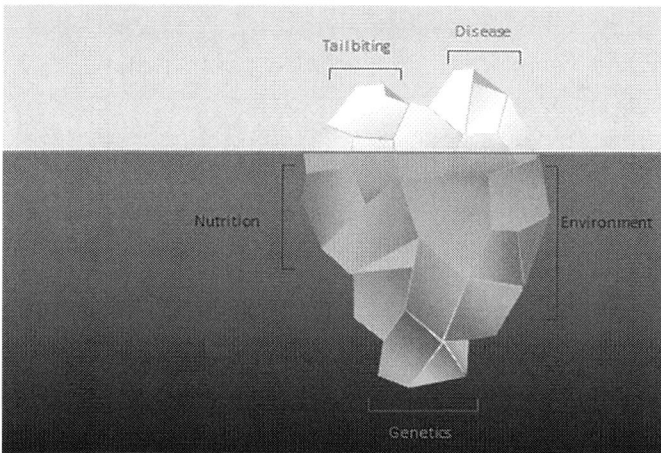

Figure 3.1 Iceberg indicators of the underlying causes.
Illustration: I. Camerlink.

3.1.1 Stereotypies

ALISTAIR B. LAWRENCE

Stereotypies are a type of 'abnormal behaviour' found in domesticated animals including farmed species. Behaviour is classed as stereotypy when it is repetitive, persistent and lacks any obvious function. Most people who have visited zoos will have seen animals, such as large carnivores, pacing around their enclosures for long periods of time usually showing great repetition in their movement patterns. In pigs, stereotypies almost always involve oral behaviours (for example, bar-biting [Figure 3.2], chain-chewing, use of the drinker and also sham-chewing) rather than locomotion, but the behaviour will again be performed over many hours of the day and be highly repetitive. The exact form of the stereotypic behaviour depends on housing (for example, sows will only be able to properly develop bar-biting if horizontal bars are available, Figure 3.2), and each sow will tend to develop its own individual pattern of stereotypy.

As the definition of stereotype implies it is not usually obvious what the animal is achieving through performing a behaviour such as bar-biting. Various suggestions have been: (1) that animals perform stereotypies because they are bored and are seeking stimulation; (2) that stereotypies allow the animal to cope with stress; (3) that stereotypies are no different to other oral behaviours, such as nosing and mouthing bedding materials. Although none of these options have been ruled out, evidence

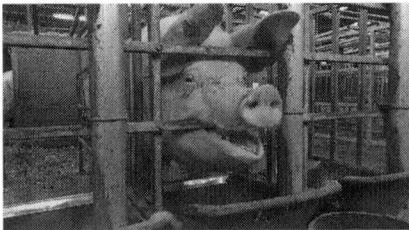

Figure 3.2 Bar-biting is one of the well known stereotypic behaviours in sows. Photo: SRUC / M. Farish.

tends towards supporting that stereotypies in pigs occur in response to high levels of arousal and stress.

While the function of stereotypic behaviours is not established it has become clear that stereotypies in pigs are often linked to restricted feeding regimes (see also Section 4.7.3 on hunger in sows). Hence, stereotypies in sows can be prevented by any of the following: increasing feeding levels, adding certain fibres (for example, sugar beet pulp) to the sows' diet or by allowing sows to express their hunger through foraging behaviours. In other words, prevention of stereotypy in sows is achieved either by reducing their hunger or by allowing sows to express their hunger. In either case stereotypies are prevented by reducing sow frustration occurring from feeding motivation. Finally, it is important to note that other stressors (for example, persistent loud noise) can exacerbate stereotypies in food-restricted sows.

3.1.2 Tail posture

MONA LILIAN VESTBJERG LARSEN AND LENE JUUL PEDERSEN

A long curly tail is often used in the media as an indicator of good welfare in pigs. However, is this really the case and does an uncurled tail indicate poor welfare? The tail of a pig can either be curled, be tucked between the hind legs or be in a posture in between, often referred to as a hanging tail. Figure 3.3 shows a pen of finisher pigs during feeding where all pigs except one have a curled tail. One pig shows the need to protect its tail during this vulnerable situation, but from what? Days-old

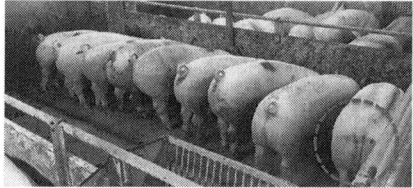

Figure 3.3 One tucked tail among curly tails. Photo: M.L.V. Larsen.

piglets tuck their tail after tail docking suggesting that a tucked tail is a sign of pain in the tail. It has also been investigated whether the tail posture of pigs changes as a reaction to tail biting, which is another painful experience.

Research has shown that a lowered tail (either tucked or hanging) can be a sign of tail damage in both weaner and finisher pigs, although tail damage is not always present and can be present on pigs without a lowered tail. Furthermore, the observation of lowered tails in a pen of weaner or finisher pigs can be an indication of tail damage developing within the next couple of days. Thus, tail posture can be used as an indicator of possible present and future tail damage in a pen of pigs. However, the tail posture of pigs seems to be not only related to pain in the tail, but perhaps also to stressors in the environment. So far, research has shown that stocking density and enrichment affect the tail posture of finisher pigs. Although, this relationship could also be caused by a higher risk of ongoing tail biting in pens with higher stocking density and in pens with a lack of proper enrichment.

Pig tail posture could be an iceberg indicator of stressful conditions, which may lead to tail biting and result in tail damage. In which case observing tail posture would increase the possibility of the farmer reacting promptly to and preventing serious tail damage as well as increasing the general welfare of the pigs. The relationship between tail posture and tail damage has only been investigated in pigs with undocked tails (such as those shown in Figure 3.3). Tail biting is a problem in both docked and undocked pigs, but with current housing conditions and management practices the prevalence of tail biting is higher when producing pigs with undocked tails. The use of tail posture as an early indicator of tail biting could ease the management when producing pigs with undocked tails. When observing tail posture, it is important to observe the pigs from outside the pen without disturbing them. This could, for example, be during feeding as seen in Figure 3.3 or through live observation or recorded video (undertaken manually or automatically).

3.1.3 Fearfulness

CÉLINE TALLET, MARIA JOSÉ HÖTZEL AND NICOLAS DEVILLERS

Fear is the reaction to a threatening event. It is a natural and adaptive behaviour that allows animals to avoid a potential danger. In the production environment, avoidance possibilities are limited or even non-existent in many situations. Thus, exposing pigs repeatedly to frightening situations may lead to chronic stress, which is detrimental to health, welfare, reproduction and productivity.

When the threat is perceived as low, pigs express vigilance reactions toward the potential danger, such as immobility, observation and opening of the ears. When the threat is perceived as high, pigs express avoidance reactions, such as moving away or trying to escape, or even defensive reactions. Escape attempts and defensive reactions can be dangerous for both pigs and their human caretakers, as both can get injured. One may not expect the same fear reaction from all pigs, as fearfulness varies among individuals. Significantly, the reaction of one fearful pig may spread to the group through behavioural signs, odours or stress vocalizations.

Several situations may be frightening for pigs. Although pigs are curious in general, unexpected or novel situations can induce fear reactions: that is, a new environment (pen or room, novel object, food or smell) or a new situation (unacquainted pig or human, new handling procedure). For example, pigs show fear during many handling procedures, such as castration, tail docking, tooth resection, vaccination, or transportation because these situations are unknown, unexpected and intense, and induce noise, pig vocalizations and agitation and sometimes pain. Isolation is especially fear eliciting because pigs are social animals.

To prevent pigs from feeling fear, handlers should reduce sources of fear as much as possible, or try to make them more familiar and less unexpected. For instance, letting piglets run in corridors of the room may help them to be less fearful when they will be moved at weaning or to the fattening pens. Treating pigs gently during routine handling is recommended; it not only decreases fear of humans, but it may help them cope better with novel environments and situations.

3.1.4 Vocalizations

CÉLINE TALLET, LISETTE M.C. LELIVELD AND ELODIE F. BRIEFER

Pigs have very good hearing capacities and are highly sensitive to frequencies corresponding to the human voice. Audition is the sense they use the most, together with olfaction. Vocalizations are thus a strong means of communication for them. As a consequence, any noise may disturb them and should be avoided. Pigs emit a large variety of sounds (grunts, squeals, squeaks, screams or even croak, chirrup or bark) that humans can hear and interpret, since they are usually produced in specific contexts. Pig calls can be classified into five types, belonging to two main categories: low-pitched and high-pitched calls.

Low-pitched (LF) calls

LF calls are expressed in both positive and negative situations and are divided into three groups.

- LF stable (low grunts), which are produced in both positive (for example, food reward) and negative contexts (for example, social isolation) with the mouth closed, but are, however, more frequent in negative situations.
- LF modulated (high grunts), which are higher pitched and produced with the mouth open. These calls are emitted in a large variety of situations (such as reunion with pen mates) and their rate may increase with the intensity of the situation.
- The last type, LF tonal, regroups croaks, chirrups and barks, which are expressed mostly in positive situations (for example, play, being with pen mates and reunion with the sow after a nursing bout).

High-pitched calls

High-pitched calls are usually expressed in negative situations and are divided into two groups.

- Screams, which are produced in highly negative situations that should be avoided whenever possible (for example, castration, crushing, pain, fighting).
- Squeals and squeaks, which are produced in less intense negative situations (for example, isolation from the group, trying to escape, unfamiliar environment).

Listening to your pigs will therefore give you insights into what is pleasant for pigs (playing, social contact), what is unpleasant (being alone, moving to unfamiliar place) and what is intolerable (pain). It could help you to adapt your management strategies, in order to improve their welfare. Nowadays, automatic systems are being developed to help you to recognize these sounds and to act accordingly (for example, STREMODO®, SOUNDWEL).

3.1.5 Tear staining

JEREMY N. MARCHANT-FORDE

Although still in the early stages of validation and application, there is evidence that tear stains may be a useful non-invasive and very obvious indicator of an individual pig's welfare state. A tear stain in the pig, is a red-brown to black facial stain seen originating from the inner corner of the eye (Figure 3.4; Table 3.1). Historically, these stains have been linked to clinical disease, such as atrophic rhinitis or poor air quality, with high ammonia and dust levels, but recent experimental studies have shown that they can be induced in clinically healthy pigs, housed in clean and sterile environments, by the application of direct stressors, and are present in on-farm pigs and related to certain welfare issues.

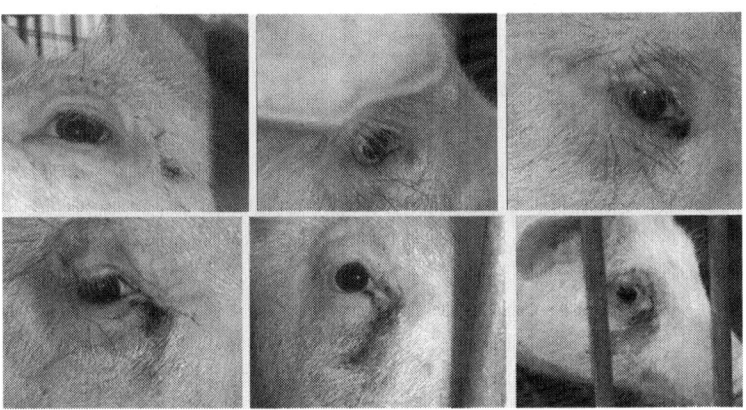

Figure 3.4 Tear staining categories in pigs, from a score 0–5. Photo: J.N. Marchant-Forde.

Table 3.1 Tear staining score.

Tear staining score (0-5)	Description
0	No signs of any staining
1	Staining is barely detectable and area stained does not extend below the eyelid
2	Staining is obvious and area stained is approximately <50% of total eye area
3	Staining is obvious and area stained is approximately 50–100% of total eye area
4	Staining is severe, area stained is approximately ≥100% of total eye area, and area stained does not extend below the mouth line
5	Staining is severe, area stained is >100% of total eye area, and area stained extends below the mouth line

The stain itself is produced by the Hardarian gland located next to the eye, which is present in most land vertebrates but absent in some species, such as humans. The gland secretes a mixture of compounds, which in some species includes pigments called porphyrins, giving the stain its distinct colour. Normally, the gland's secretions have photoprotective and possible immune functions.

Experimentally, tear staining has been shown to be related to sympathetic nervous system activation (flight or fight response) and is higher in pigs housed in isolation and without access to enrichment. In on-farm studies, larger stains have been shown to be related to lower social status, lack of access to enrichment and increased tail damage from tail biting. Pigs with larger stains are also slower to approach novel objects placed in the pen, demonstrating more fearfulness. Stains are also bigger in castrated male pigs compared to females, and in sows whose litters do not have access to enrichment.

Within an on-farm population, there will be a general level of staining present, but superimposed on this will be variation. Pigs with very pronounced stains of 4 or 5 on the 0–5 scale should be rare (Figure 3.4; Table 3.1), but should be inspected thoroughly, to identify any welfare or health issues that may be present.

3.1.6 Skin lesions at slaughter

NIENKE VAN STAAVEREN

While it is important to observe pigs on your farm, it can be difficult to measure skin lesions when pigs are dirty, moving around a lot or when lighting is poor. For these reasons, skin lesions can also be measured at slaughter. Skin lesions at slaughter (as in Figure 3.5) are suggested as iceberg indicators, meaning that they reflect different aspects of a pig's life, such as aggressive interactions and mounting behaviour, but also other welfare issues, such as poor body condition, bursitis, huddling or coughing in the weaner or finisher stages. In fact, skin lesions on the carcass can reflect lesions that were received at least 10 weeks earlier. Skin lesions are not routinely recorded at the abattoir in all countries, although in some countries, such as Denmark, the Netherlands and the UK, they are being recorded to improve health, welfare and productivity by reporting this information back to farmers. Farmers could use this information to benchmark their farm over time or against other farmers and, if needed, to improve on-farm management practices that could contribute to welfare issues associated with skin lesions observed at the abattoir.

Skin lesions can be scored according to severity of the 'scratches' using different scoring systems or by counting the number of lesions on different parts of the body. It is important to remember that skin lesions can occur in different phases of a pig's life. The age of the lesions can be used to distinguish lesions occurring on the farm (older lesions with scabs) from lesions that happened during transport or lairage (fresher lesions). Also, if a similar pattern of lesions or bruising is found on pig carcasses from different farmers, it is likely that this occurred in the abattoir. Abattoir processes, such as scalding and dehairing, typically increase the visibility of skin lesions though it might mask more mild skin lesions. Abattoir processes can also cause some damage to the carcass, but this is easily distinguishable from real skin lesions due to their pale appearance and should be recorded separately.

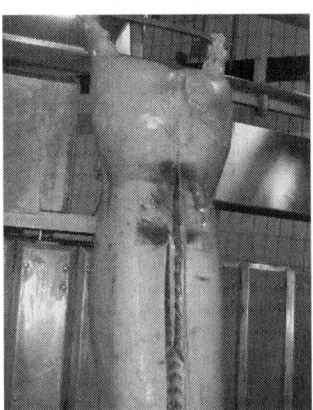

Figure 3.5 Bruising of the carcass at slaughter. Photo: Teagasc/L. Boyle.

3.2 Welfare assessment methods

ANTONIO VELARDE CALVO AND ANTONI DALMAU

Welfare comprises physical and mental health and includes freedom from thirst or hunger, from discomfort, from disease, pain and injuries, from fear and distress, and the freedom to express normal behaviour, referred to as the Five Freedoms (FAWC, 1992). The Welfare Quality® protocol offers a standardized method, scientifically sound and feasible, to assess animal welfare on commercial conditions. The protocol is built on the Five Freedoms and was designed with the expertise of researchers across Europe. It has formed the basis of many other assessment protocols for pigs and other farm animals. It considers 4 principles and 12 criteria, as shown in Table 3.2. The specific measures for sows with piglets and for growing pigs are given in the Appendices.

Table 3.2 Welfare Quality® principles and criteria.

Principle	Welfare criteria	
Good feeding	1	Absence of prolonged hunger
	2	Absence of prolonged thirst
Good housing	3	Comfort around resting
	4	Thermal comfort
	5	Ease of movement
Good health	6	Absence of injuries
	7	Absence of disease
	8	Absence of pain induced by management procedures

Table 3.2 *continued*

Principle	Welfare criteria
Appropriate behaviour	9 Expression of social behaviours
	10 Expression of other behaviours
	11 Good human–animal relationship
	12 Positive emotional state

3.2.1 Resource- versus animal-based measures

Traditionally, monitoring systems and legislation largely relied on examination of resource- and management-based measures (also referred to as 'input' or 'design' measures). These measures consider 'what' or 'how much' different resources are given to animals (that is, pens design, space requirements and so on). These parameters are easy to define, to measure and have a high repeatability. However, these measures have often been criticized for potentially low validity due largely to unpredictable outcomes. Animals may experience the same situation or handling procedure differently depending of their genetic background, temperament, previous experiences or just luck.

The emphasis of the Welfare Quality® protocols is placed on animal-based measures (also called 'outcome' or 'performance' measures) in an attempt to estimate the actual welfare state of animals in terms of, for instance, their behaviour, fearfulness, health or physical condition. Such measures have inherent advantages over resource-based measures. Animal-based measures are likely to be the most direct reflection of their welfare state. It permits welfare evaluation through direct observation of the animal, regardless of how and where it is kept. As it is applicable to all farms, animal-based measures permit comparisons of animals' welfare from different places, systems and countries, and remain more transparent to stakeholders. Resource- and management-based measures can be used to complement the animal-based measures when there are no promising animal-based measures available. Moreover, resource measures can also be used to identify risks to animal welfare and to identify causes of poor welfare so that improvement strategies can be implemented. For example, if tail biting is found in a farm, environmental indicators (such as enrichment material, feed composition or temperatures) will be checked to solve the problem.

3.2.2 The Welfare Quality® protocol in practice

The welfare assessment should be carried out in accordance with the published protocols (examples provided at the Appendices) (Welfare Quality®, 2009). The assessment involves collecting data on both animals and resources. A specific order is provided in the protocol for the measures to be taken on farms for each animal type. In general, the animal-based assessment starts with measures recorded from outside the pen and by observing the whole group. In sows and growing pigs, for example, the measures recorded from outside the pen consist of those related to the positive emotional state criterion (by means of the Qualitative Behavioural Assessment (Section 3.3), the expression of social and other behaviours (scan sampling), and the presence of stereotypies, respiratory problems (coughing and sneezing) and thermal comfort measures (shivering, panting, huddling). Afterwards, the assessor enters the pen to assess the human–animal relationship and other animal-based measures related to the welfare principles of good feeding, housing and health. Animals are individually scored for body condition, bursitis, shoulder sores, dirtiness (or presence of manure on the body), wounds on the body, tail biting, vulva lesions, lameness, pumping (heavy and laboured breathing), twisted snouts, rectal prolapse, uterine prolapse, skin condition, constipation, scouring, metritis, mastitis, local infections, tremor, splay leg and hernias. These measures are taken in approximately 30 pregnant sows, in 10 lactating sows and their litters, and/or in 150 growing pigs from 10 different pens. Some measures will require sampling of animals at specific stages of pregnancy (early, mid and late gestation) or at different stages of the growing/fattening period. Rather than entering many different pens and selecting lots of different animals the same animals should be used for as many different measures as possible to save time and minimize disturbance. On many farms, animals in different stages may be housed within the same building (or even room), and are likely to be distributed equally across the building/room.

The Welfare Quality® assessment protocols are readily available but they alone do not guarantee effective assessment; meaningful data can only be obtained when observers in each country have the same level of training. To standardize the implementation of the assessment protocol and achieve high repeatability between assessors, they must be continuously assessed during a robust training course until they develop a uniform scoring.

3.2.3 Other welfare assessment methods

Research studies often use physiological indicators related to the stress response to assess welfare. These can include heart rate, respiratory rate, body temperature and plasma levels of glucocorticoids. When an animal is stressed, for example, by experiencing anxiety or uncertainty, the brain releases adrenocorticotropic hormone, which stimulates the adrenal gland to release glucocorticoids within minutes of the event. When this state of stress is maintained over a longer time, this chronic stress can be detected by increased cortisol levels in the pigs' hair. Physiological measures might not be feasible on commercial conditions due to the need for experimental equipment or laboratory analyses in addition to the behavioural tests.

References

FAWC (1992) Farm Animal Welfare Council updates the five freedoms. *Veterinary Record* 131(17), 357.

Welfare Quality (2009) Welfare Quality® assessment protocol for pigs (sows and piglets, growing and finishing pigs). Welfare Quality® Consortium, Lelystad, the Netherlands. Available at: http://www.welfarequality.net/media/1018/pig_protocol.pdf (accessed 6 July 2019).

3.3 Qualitative behaviour assessment

FRANÇOISE WEMELSFELDER

Qualitative behaviour assessment (QBA) is a method that is frequently used in research to study animal emotions, and has been included in various EU welfare assessment protocols. Veterinarians or auditors may use a QBA scoring protocol, but you can also do this yourself. Applying QBA regularly to pigs in various age groups will give an impression of their emotional well-being, and may alert farmers to welfare concerns within these groups.

3.3.1 Learning to see how pigs feel

Pigs are smart, sensitive animals with personalities, feelings and thoughts. They can remember things for a long time, and can out-perform dogs and chimpanzees in intelligence tests. Taking an interest in pigs' perspective on the world, and considering their point of view, is crucial to improve their welfare. One way to do this is to observe the expressive body language that pigs show when moving around. Pigs do not just walk, eat, sit, or lie down mechanically, they always do such things in a certain way, with a certain style of movement, which reveals how they experience a situation (Figure 3.6). They can be relaxed, at ease, playful and curious, or, by contrast, tense, scared and depressed.

Such terms describe different emotional qualities of pigs' body language, whether observed individually or as a group. Such qualities can over-lap and vary together in many different ways; a pig can be confident in a calm or excited way, and be calm in a relaxed or tense way. What

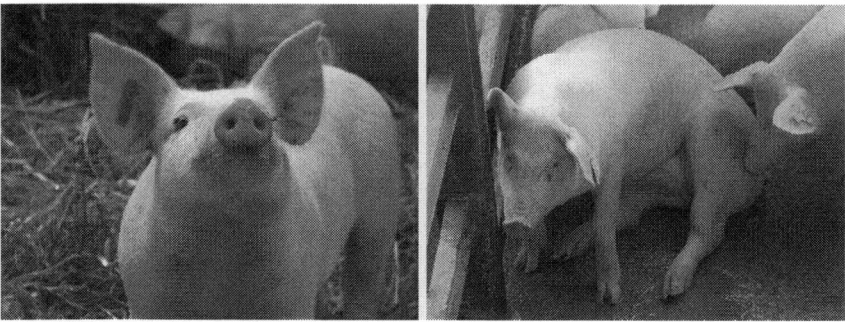

Figure 3.6 Pigs can show clear body language. Photo: SRUC/M. Farish.

matters is that you learn to recognize *patterns* of expression and understand their importance for welfare. Pigs might show fear for a moment, but if they appear relaxed and at ease most of the time this is not a problem for welfare; if, however, they seem chronically tense and irritable, that is a problem needing attention.

3.3.2 Reading pigs is a skill

If you spend time with your pigs and develop a sense for their body language, it will be easier to care for their well-being. In fact, this is a traditional skill; farmers who know their animals well can spot problems at an early stage, avoiding worsening of the problem (Section 4.1). Several sections in this book mention the importance of reading body language for managing welfare (Sections 3.1.2, 3.1.5, 4.1), and so developing this skill will bring a range of benefits.

QBA is a method well suited to this. Its most important principle is that you must closely observe how the whole animal moves. The position of body parts such as ears and tail are an important aspect of body language (Section 3.1.2), but it is the *whole* animal's posture and way of subtly moving those body parts that conveys how it is actually feeling. For example, when pigs are resting, the difference between relaxed contentment and uneasy boredom may not be easy to spot, but there will be telling expressive clues such as tension and restlessness. However, if you see the same pigs every day, you may become desensitized to such clues. It is good therefore to visit farms where pigs have different amounts of space, outdoor access and environmental stimulation, and to compare how this affects the pigs' expressions. This should give you a better understanding of the condition of your own pigs.

3.3.3 How to use QBA

QBA works by asking people to score 15 to 20 terms describing an animal's body language. The EU Welfare Quality® protocol for pigs (Section 3.2) contains a list of 10 positive and 10 negative QBA terms.

Active	Playful	Tense
Relaxed	Positively occupied	Frustrated
Calm	Lively	Bored
Content	Happy	Listless
Enjoying	Fearful	Indifferent
Sociable	Agitated	Irritable
Aimless	Distressed	

Each of these terms is scored on an unstructured rating scale, ranging from 'not at all', to 'could not be more', as in the example below. So, ask yourself 'how relaxed are these pigs', or 'how frustrated', and place a tick on the scale for these terms in between 'not at all' and 'could not be more', to mark the intensity of the pigs' expression.

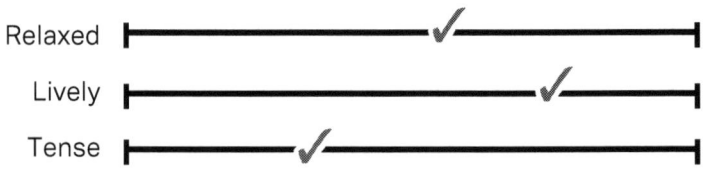

Doing this for all 20 terms gives you quite a comprehensive, nuanced picture of how pigs are feeling. If you would score a range of different pig herds, a pattern would emerge showing how these pigs differ in their overall expressive profile. Most of the time, as the Figure 3.7 illustrates, profiles vary along two dimensions (mood and energy), that together form four quadrants: positive energetic expression (for example, playful), positive low energy expression (for example, chilled), negative energetic expression (for example, frustrated) and negative low energy expression (for example, indifferent). The scientific literature tends to label these dimensions as 'valence' (mood) and 'arousal' (energy).

To try QBA for yourself, closely observe your pigs at different times of day, and then use the scoring list to estimate in which quadrant(s) they appear to be located. You can do this using the app when it becomes available (Section 3.5), or using the scoring list in the appendix. Looking at the pigs' overall expressive profile, how often are they happily engaged with their surroundings and each other, and how often

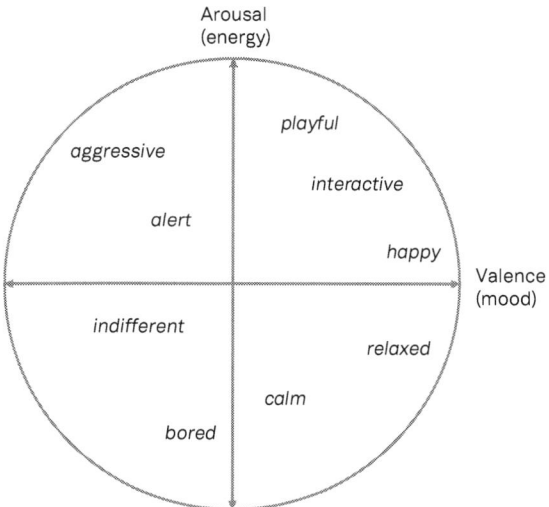

Figure 3.7 An example of an expressive QBA profile along mood and energy dimensions. Illustration: SRUC/F. Wemelsfelder.

aimlessly wandering around, looking for something to do? How often do they appear settled and relaxed, and how often nervous and aggressive? And, following up such observations, what can you do to improve the pigs' conditions and increase their positive expressivity and emotional well-being?

3.3.4 Using QBA to improve welfare

Practicing QBA will enhance your awareness of pigs' emotional well-being, but will not tell you *why* pigs are feeling a certain way. There could be one or many causes, with short- or long-term impacts. It is therefore important to experiment with making small changes and to observe the effect they have on the pigs – this book provides many suggestions for what you could do (Section 4.9). One of QBA's strengths is that it is particularly useful for addressing positive expressions of welfare, and not merely whether animals are suffering or not. When pigs are given positive opportunities to enjoy life (Section 4.2), this will increase a farmer's work satisfaction too. QBA could be an easy, cost-free, and rewarding way of engaging with the animals on your farm.

3.4 Precision farming for automatic detection of welfare risks

Historically farmers managed livestock and took care of animal welfare on the basis of audio-visual observation performed on a routine basis. Nowadays, the size of livestock farms rapidly increases and the number of animals that the farmer has to observe and manage is much higher than in the past. A consequence of these changes is, for example, that in the Netherlands a farmer has on average 1 second per day for observing a fattening pig in a modern, industrial farm. In addition, the supply of stockworkers with the necessary management skills is limited and the profit margins of livestock farming are slim. These factors create new risks for pig welfare as the farmer might not notice when problems occur.

3.4.1 Precision livestock farming (PLF)

The development of new, sensor-based tools supports farmers and increases their sensory modalities (providing additional ways to observe animals, for example, by infra-red thermography). Modern technology enables the use of sensors, such as cameras or microphones, to supplement farmers' eyes and ears in monitoring animals at shed, compartment, pen or even individual levels.

A major advantage of sensor-based monitoring is its continuous character. This means that monitoring can be always on, 7 days a week, 24 hours a day. This is clearly advantageous if we compare this to the time that the farmer can manually observe animals in industrial husbandry systems. Thus, continuous monitoring brings the animals closer to the farmer, especially in industrial systems, where contact between the individual animal and the farmer is very limited. The farmer can obtain insight about the animal and its welfare, thanks to sensor technology, which is not possible on the basis of short lasting, personal audio-visual observation. Thus, the farmer can invest their time in the animals that require attention. Moreover, welfare assessment methods such as Welfare Quality® protocol can only be carried out sporadically, which is not sufficient to deal with problems happening in real-time.

Early PLF developments were mainly initiated by the European research community. Early adopters are starting to use PLF systems, mainly in Europe, despite the fact that the PLF concept is rather new in the European pig industry. So far there is a lack of products on the market that comprehensively approach pig welfare monitoring. However, there are already systems available that allow monitoring of individual indicators of pig welfare, such as water or feed consumption or weight. There are several advantages of PLF technology that will lead to its wider adoption in the coming years.

3.4.2 Monitoring water consumption

One example of PLF systems in which the continuous character of monitoring is especially important is water consumption. Water consumption monitoring is a very simple and cost-effective tool for recording changes in water drinking patterns, which are directly related to health and welfare. Currently on most pig farms water consumption is not monitored. In the best case, malfunctioning drinkers are detected by regular checks. This is obviously not sufficient as in many cases malfunctioning of a water supply is detected only when animals are already deprived from water for a prolonged time, showing up in behavioural or health problems. Continuous monitoring detects and allows intervention before animals are affected.

3.4.3 Treating respiratory problems effectively

PLF systems offer real-time monitoring and this allows for immediate responses to welfare problems. Respiratory diseases are a welfare problem in which real-time response is crucial. Respiratory diseases negatively affect average daily gain, feed conversion rate and homogeneity of pig weight. To minimize these negative effects pigs should be treated as soon as possible when a disease is detected.

The Belgian start-up company Soundtalks developed an automated system that is based on microphones. The system registers sounds in a pig compartment and then detects illness-related coughs. Monitoring pig coughs with microphones in real-time allows early detection of respiratory diseases. This makes it possible to treat animals at an early stage of disease, which reduces a risk of further outbreaks, costs of treatment and it improves pig welfare.

3.4.4 Information supply

For most farmers, the volume of water consumed or the number of coughs in a compartment is less relevant than an explicit alarm indicating that water consumption is too low or that pigs have respiratory problems. In order to be useful for the farmer, PLF systems aim to provide processed information based on which the farmer can take action. This means that raw sensor data is first modelled to select relevant information and only then are these models used in real-time for monitoring and control purposes. Through the provision of useful information to skilled stockworkers, manual monitoring can be automatized by modern sensor technology.

Alongside the advantages and promises PLF technology application has for pig welfare monitoring there are also risks of which farmers should be aware. PLF solutions are in early stages of development and legal regulations on the application of these technologies did not exist until 2019. This also means that there are no formalized PLF standards to which companies developing such systems have to adhere. The consequence is that when investing in PLF systems farmers are forced to trust the company offering a product. Without scientific and independent validation, the risk of investment is entirely on the farmer. This situation is comparable to human health monitoring with wearables (such as smart watches) where only a small percentage of devices (5%) are scientifically validated.

3.5 Animal welfare apps

IRENE CAMERLINK

Based on the various welfare assessment methods some smartphone apps have been developed as part of research projects. Although the apps may have limited availability depending on software system or target group (restricted access with password), may currently not be in English or may not be continued over the course of time, it is likely that more of these apps will become accessible in future. Best is to ask on national level if there are any tools available. The apps are often designed for welfare assessors or farmers and are user friendly. Note, however, that any app is a guiding tool and gives an indication of the welfare. In the development of a Slovenian app to reduce tail biting, a pig farmer rightly concluded that it is essential that the app is filled in honestly and precisely in order to benefit from its results. Still, outcomes should not be taken as hard evidence for the actual welfare situation. For a proper welfare assessment consult an assessor of one of the assurance schemes or your veterinarian.

3.5.1 Qualitative behaviour assessment

The original developers of the QBA method are in the process of developing a user-friendly, web-based QBA application with advice and training functions that anyone interested in scoring pig body language could use. In the meantime, what you can do is closely observe your pigs at different times of day, and ask in which quadrant(s) you think they are located. How often are they happily engaged with their surroundings and each other, and how often aimlessly wandering around, looking for something to do? How often do they appear settled and relaxed, and how often nervous and aggressive? And, most importantly, what can you do to improve the pigs' conditions and increase their positive expressivity and emotional well-being?

3.5.2 Ferkel Indikatoren Check

German-speaking countries can make use of an app to score welfare of piglets. Ferkel Indikatoren Check 4+ (Land24 GmbH, Germany) is available only for iOS devices. It is freely available and can be downloaded in the App Store.

The app guides you through a roughly 2 hour farm check to find the strong and weak points of the farm and points for improvement.

3.5.3 Veescan voor varkens

For Dutch farmers there is the 'Veescan voor varkens', developed by De Boerenbond/ILVO. It is freely available in the Play Store and App Store. The app is based on the Five Freedoms for animal welfare, which is also the basis for the Welfare Quality® protocol. After completing the app, you receive a report with a welfare score and information on potential risk factors. By completing the questions in the app more frequently you can track the progress made.

3.5.6 Varkens app

The Dutch 'Varkens app' (Android and iOS) includes a book on pig husbandry including management, physiology, nutrition and health. It also includes information on pig prices.

3.6 Know the welfare of your pigs

IRENE CAMERLINK

You can assess welfare at your farm using one of the available protocols (given in appendices). Here is a shortened version to make a brief initial assessment or to re-evaluate scores after changes in management have been made. This scoring form can be used for growing pigs.

The body condition score of 1–5 relates to the scores that are also used for sows, with:

1 = emaciated
2 = thin
3 = ideal
4 = fat
5 = overly fat.

The score of 0, 1, 2 relates to the percentage of pigs in the group seen with the indicated measure.

0 = the measure is largely absent in the group
1 = it is occurring in about 20% of the group
2 = it is occurring in more than 20% of the group.

Simplified scoring table			
0: largely absent; 1: occurring in up to 20% of group; 2: occurring in >20% of group			
PART 1			
Criteria	Measure	Score (circle answer)	Write remarks
Hunger	Body condition score	1 2 3 4 5	
Thirst	# *working* drinkers?	Good / Sufficient / Poor	
	Are drinkers clean?	Good / Sufficient / Poor	
Resting	Injuries from lying	0 1 2	
	Manure on body	0 1 2	
Thermal comfort	Panting	0 1 2	
	Huddling, shivering	0 1 2	
Movement	Space allowance	m² / pig	
Injuries	Lameness	0 1 2	
	Wounds	0 1 2	
	Tail lesions	0 1 2	
Disease	Coughing	0 1 2	
	Diarrhoea	0 1 2	
Procedures	Castration	Yes / No	
	Tail docking	Yes / No	
	Teeth grinding	Yes / No	

Simplified scoring table			
PART 2			
Criteria	Measure	Enter frequency, time and circle terms	Score (circle answer)
Social behaviours + exploration	Tally positive, negative, social and explorative behaviour for 5 minutes (10 second/ animal)	Positive (play, body contact):	Mostly positive
			Mostly negative
		Negative (fighting, biting, head knocks):	Mostly neutral
		Social neutral (nose contact):	
		Exploration (rooting, chewing, nosing environment):	0 1 2
Fear of humans	How quick do they approach? Step in the pen and measure the time.	Time until first approach:	Mostly curious
			Mostly reluctant
		Time until first touch:	Mostly avoidant
Expression	Mark the terms that best describe the group body language	active fearful agitated frustrated aimless happy bored lively calm playful content relaxed distressed sociable enjoying tense	Mostly positive
			Mostly negative
			Mostly neutral

CHAPTER 4

What you can do to improve animal welfare?

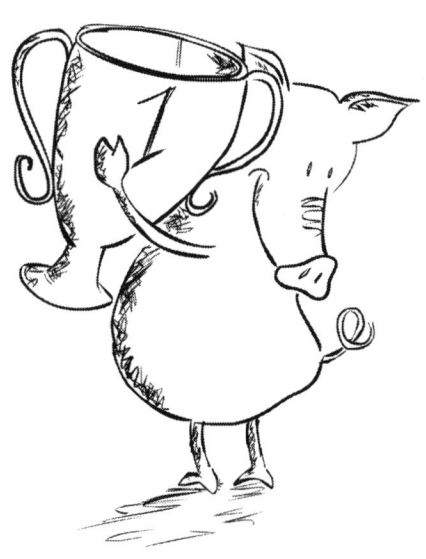

4.1 Improving human–animal interactions

JEREMY M. SKUSE, JEAN-LOUP RAULT AND PAUL HEMSWORTH

Human behaviour can have important and long-lasting effects on the welfare of pigs and their productivity. Sows that are highly fearful of humans produce on average 6% less pigs weaned per year than sows that showed low levels of fear towards humans. Similarly, highly fearful grower pigs show on average a 7% reduction in growth compared to those with lower fear of humans. Hence, the aim is to reduce fear of humans in pigs, and to develop and cultivate a positive human–animal relationship.

Research carried out in pig farms worldwide revealed that a high percentage of pigs are fearful of humans (see Table 4.1 with data from ProHand Pigs®). Figure 4.1 depicts the amount of time and effort (measured by number of slaps and pushes) that it takes to move pigs along an unfamiliar route. As you can see, highly fearful pigs took more time and effort to move compared to pigs with low fear levels.

Table 4.1 Fear of humans between farms.

Fear of humans	Percentage of farms
High fear	24%
Moderate fear	35%
Low fear	41%

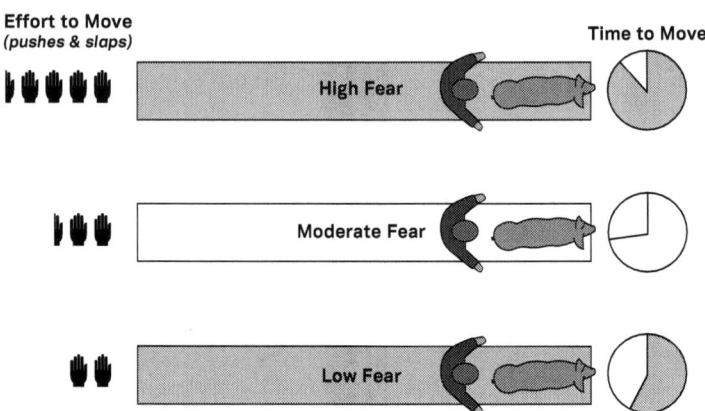

Figure 4.1 Relationship between fear of humans and handling. Illustration: ProHand Pigs®.

We are not talking about making pets out of your pigs, but if you can reduce the fear level of the pigs, they will be easier to handle and consequently be quicker to move. This will reduce the risk of injury to both you and the pig, and their welfare and productivity will be improved.

4.1.1 Assessing the human–pig relationship

It is relatively simple to test the quality of the human–pig relationship. First, stand outside the pen and assess the pigs' approach to you: reach with your arm inside the pen towards the pigs and count how many pigs approach and the latency to touch you. Remember that pigs can be hesitant to approach a standing human, so squatting down to their level makes it less scary. Pigs are very curious animals and it usually does not take long before they approach and touch the person, clothes and boots. Second, step into the pen and slowly approach a specific pig at one step per second. Write down at what approximate distance you were from the pig when it started moving, or whether you were able to touch the pig without it withdrawing. Pigs that are not fearful of humans should have low to no avoidance distance. These tests are quick to perform and do not require any specific tool. If conducted in a standardized manner, these tests provide a good idea about how pigs perceive the human. It can be useful to repeat these tests at different ages, with different batches of pigs or after specific interventions to detect changes in the human–pig relationship.

4.1.2 Negative interactions

It is important to remember that pigs are curious and sensitive animals. They are sensitive to noise, pain, temperature, overcrowding, unexpected changes in the environment and, especially, our behaviour.

Research has clearly shown that stockpeople who have fearful pigs mainly use negative behaviours, such as hits, slaps, kicks and pushes, when handling their animals. Therefore, the reason that pigs are fearful is that they learn to associate the stockperson with these negative behaviours, and as a result become fearful of humans. Pigs can discriminate between different humans, and remember whether this person interacted with them in a positive or negative manner for at least 5 weeks. When a pig is handled by several stockpeople however, the pig's fear level will be determined by the overall balance of positive and negative behaviours. Therefore, it is important that every stockperson is positive toward the pigs.

The effect of handling is often underestimated. For instance, the time that a piglet is handled during processing causes at least as much distress as the various procedures applied to the pig (for example teeth clipping, iron injection and so on).

Negative behaviours that cause fear does not only mean the obvious kick or hit, but also moderate negative behaviours, such as a slap, when used frequently. A moderate slap is a negative behaviour when the slap is applied with enough force that it can be clearly heard. Thus, moderate negative behaviours that frighten or startle pigs also contribute to the development of high fear levels in pigs.

4.1.3 Tips to reduce stress

- Use handling aids, such as 'pig boards', to move pigs quietly and swiftly but do not hit or slap pigs with these aids.
- Minimize restraint.
- Never handle a pig by pulling its ear or its tail.
- Avoid the use of electric goads and other devices that cause pain and distress.
- Use a calm voice. Avoid shouting or other forms of loud noise as it alarms the pigs.
- Do use cues, such as by knocking on the door before entering the room, so that pigs are aware that a person is coming and they are not startled.
- Moving pigs in small groups generally facilitates ease of movement and the need for negative behaviours.

It is necessary to occasionally use some negative behaviours when moving pigs. However, it is inappropriate and counter-productive to use negative behaviours more often than is necessary. It is equally important to use positive behaviours when the opportunity arises.

4.1.4 Positive interactions

A positive human–pig relationship is more than just a welfare benefit, as many studies show that it also results in pigs that are easier to handle, calmer, and in turn, these pigs contribute to better working condition and improved job satisfaction for the stockperson. Research has shown that stockpeople who use mainly positive behaviours such as pats, strokes, a hand resting on the pig's back, quiet talking, and slow deliberate movement, have pigs with the lowest fear levels.

Even brief contacts can have long-lasting effects on the human–pig relationship. Research has shown that scratching sows for just 15 seconds a day behind the ears improved the human–pig relationship. Pigs like

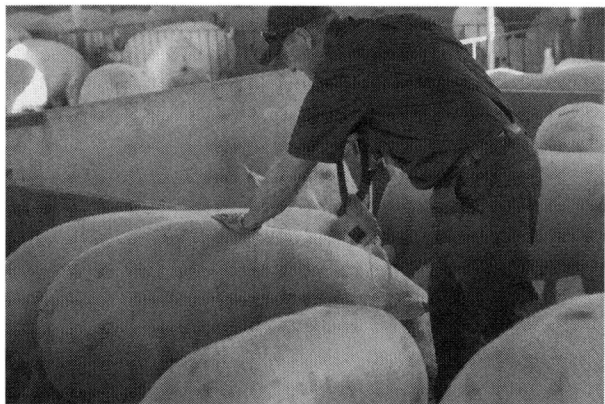

Figure 4.2 Positive interaction with a sow following vaccination. Photo: J. Skuse.

to be scratched on their neck and back (not their ears), as it is harder for them to scratch this body part themselves. They also enjoy belly rubs once they trust the human. Even management practices that are negative to pigs, like receiving a vaccination shot, can be turned into a positively perceived event if the human combines it with a gentle stroke or scratch during or after performing the procedure (Figure 4.2).

It is important to start building a positive relationship when the pigs are young (see Section 4.9 on gilt rearing). For instance, stroking piglets during sucking bouts on the first day of life led to less struggling and escape attempts when the piglets were later processed, and reduced fear weeks later.

4.1.5 Tips to improve the human–pig relationship:

- Move slowly and avoid sudden movement.
- Allow pigs to approach you and interact.
- Use gentle tactile contacts: pats, strokes, hand resting on the pigs' back.
- Talk in a quiet voice.

- Talk to the pigs to let them know you are present as they might not be able to see you.
- Walk the pens daily, this will assist the pigs to become familiar with humans.

Improving the human–animal relationship is easy to achieve, requires little time and effort, and no extra tools, and is likely to result in low fear of humans in pigs. Hence, it is a simple but good return on investment, given all the potential benefits mentioned above. Your behaviour towards pigs is crucial and plays an important role in determining their overall welfare and productivity. By maximizing your positive behaviour and minimizing your negative behaviour, you can make a big difference!

Recommended sources

Grandin, T. (2003) Best practices for handling pigs: a DVD slideshow. From *Handling of Pigs*. Grandin Livestock Handling System, Inc., Colorado, US. www.grandin.com.

Hemsworth, P. and Coleman, G. (2010) *Human-livestock Interactions: The Stockperson and the Productivity and Welfare of Intensively Farmed Animals*, 2nd edn., Wallingford: CABI.

ProHand®, an original concept developed by Australian Pork Limited and the Animal Welfare Science Centre in 1996. https://aussiepigfarmers.com.au/people/our-training/prohand/

4.2 Appropriate enrichment

HELEEN A. VAN DE WEERD

Environmental enrichment is a term used to describe a modification to the living environment of an animal. Enrichment aims to enhance living conditions and to improve the welfare of animals by enabling species-specific behaviours. In pigs, it enhances barren living conditions and provides an outlet for the need to explore. It is also a tool to manage behaviours, such as tail biting.

4.2.1 Principles of effective enrichment

Pigs in nature spend much of their time foraging and rooting. Farmed pigs largely lack the possibility to express their need to explore their environment and to forage (sniffing, biting and chewing). If pigs cannot perform these behaviours, they can become bored and frustrated with the associated risk of undesirable behaviour, such as tail and ear biting. Enrichment for pigs needs to meet specific characteristics, such as being chewable (Figure 4.3) in order to be effective. All of the characteristics listed in Table 4.2 need to be present in each enrichment material for pigs.

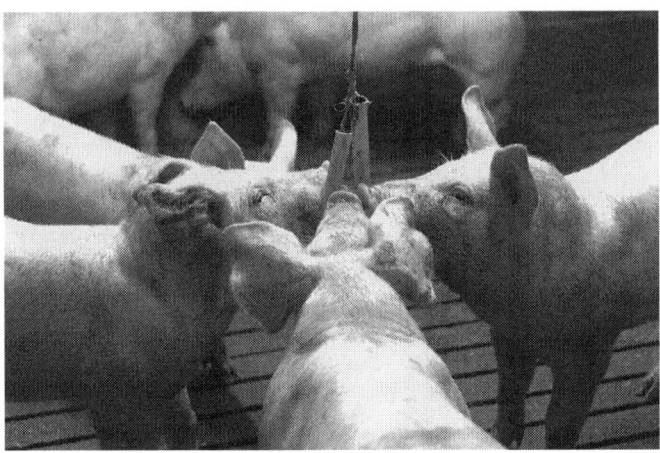

Figure 4.3 Pigs with a chewable toy. Photo: World Animal Protection.

Table 4.2 The main characteristics of effective pig enrichment

Main characteristic	So that pigs can	Provided in such a way that it
Investigable	Explore the material with their nose (rooting) and mouth	Remains interesting to a pig (by providing sufficient quantities)
Manipulable	Change the material's location, appearance and structure	Is accessible by suspending it at eye or floor level
Chewable (deformable, destructible)	Manipulate the material by biting and chewing	Is accessible for oral manipulation by all/most pigs in the pen
Edible (with an interesting texture, flavour or smell)	Ingest (eat) the material (that has some nutritional value) Note: regular feed is not regarded as enrichment	Is clean, safe and hygienic (minimising the risks of injury or contamination with chemicals or disease-causing agents)

4.2.2 Choice of enrichment

The most effective enrichment for pigs is substrate bedding as it fulfils all the key characteristics shown in Table 4.2. Slatted floors and manure systems may make it difficult to provide substrate bedding. Although there are enrichment materials that are compatible with slurry and slatted floor systems (for example, long chopped straw, Lucerne/alfalfa and hemp). In some areas, substrates may not be available, the climate may be too hot (and humid) or biosecurity may prevent the use of substrates. In these situations, small amounts of suitable substrates can be provided in racks, dispensers or trays (Figure 4.4).

A substrate rack can be installed on a slatted floor if a plate is put underneath to collect any fallen substrate. In order to to keep the substrate clean and reduce undesirable behaviour such as oral manipulations of pen mates around 400 g/day of substrate should be provided per pig.

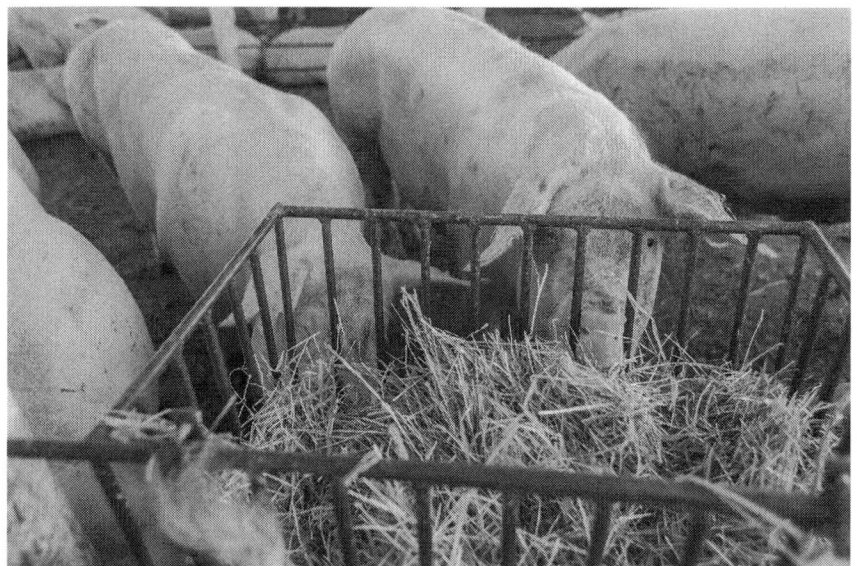

Figure 4.4 Sows at a hay rack. Photo: World Animal Protection/N. Castro.

Point-source objects are an alternative, but many of the available objects do not meet the above criteria and pigs easily loose interest. The most common (non-effective) enrichment objects are (car) tyres, metal chains and simple plastic objects. These objects are not useful or interesting, and can be associated with hazards (for example, metal wire in tyres, breakable plastics, chewing on metal can cause tooth and gum damage). Another common error is objects being presented wrongly, for example, objects are offered on the floor, but after a short period of use, end up in a corner of a pen or get stuck under a feeder (not available anymore) and become soiled with manure (a health hazard).

TIP 1

Owing to their anatomy, pigs cannot raise their heads much higher than back level. Therefore, hanging objects should not be above eye level.

Effective enrichment is different for different age groups and needs to be adjusted to their needs at that time (Table 4.3).

Table 4.3

Type of pig	Specific considerations for enrichment
Growing/ fattening pigs and gilts	It is important to make sure that individual dominant pigs cannot prevent other pigs from using (point-source) enrichment objects. For (bought in) gilts that arrive newly on a farm, providing (edible substrate) enrichment can be a means of habituating them to human presence which will benefit handling.
Breeding or teaser boars	Boars can destroy materials quickly. The easiest form of enrichment is to provide a substrate bedding.

Type of pig	Specific considerations for enrichment
Gestation sows	Breeding sows are fed a restricted diet, which means that they are very highly motivated to find food. It is therefore beneficial to address some of that hunger and the need to forage and chew with suitable enrichment. This can be done by providing substrates that will address these strong motivations and allow them to ingest some fibre.
Lactating sows	The enrichment provided needs to function within the restricted environment of the farrowing crate. The most suitable materials are substrates provided at the head of the sow, or burlap sacks (jute) or ropes on the side of the crate that the sow can reach.
Piglets (before and after weaning)	Enrichment will need to be adjusted to the size of the piglets, and extra attention needs to be paid to biosecurity. Objects need to be large enough to allow multiple piglets to use it, in a similar way as synchronized suckling.

4.2.3 What is enough?

A common mistake is that only one enrichment object is provided for a group of pigs. This may cause competition and frustration, expressed as aggression or tail biting. Fights may not necessarily happen close to the provided objects. When new objects are provided most pigs in the group will want to explore it. The same issue is with small enrichment objects that allow only a limited number of pigs to interact with it simultaneously. If more than one pig can play with an object then this enhances the interest in an object.

Enrichment should allow as many active pigs as possible with the opportunity to use the enrichment. Ideally, about 85–100% of active pigs should be able to interact with enrichment.

TIP 2

Use the score forms at the end of the book to calculate if you provide enough and correct enrichment.

4.2.4 Renewal rate

The frequency of enrichment renewal, to keep pigs interested, depends on the type of material provided. Substrate bedding needs to be topped up to stay fresh.

Pigs retain a memory of objects and interactions and it is therefore recommended to have a regular rotation of point-source objects between pens, in which a minimum of 5 days elapses before they have same object. Some farms use an overhead system with wires and wheels from which enrichment objects hang, that can be easily moved to hang over another pen.

Sharing enrichment items on a rotational basis between pens could be a potential biosecurity risk, which can be overcome with cleaning and disinfection procedures for all re-usable enrichment items. Additionally, all enrichment items should be checked regularly to ensure they have no sharp edges or breakable pieces that could be chewed and ingested, potentially causing obstruction or injury.

4.2.5 Where to place enrichment

Enrichment material must be accessible to all pigs at all times. In pens with high animal densities there are often no clear functional areas for activity and sleeping. In group pens with sequential feeding stations where pigs take turns to eat it is easier to identify the areas for activity (around the feeder) and for resting and sleeping (solid floor areas).

As a general rule, enrichment objects should be provided close to (but not in) the areas that are used for eating, drinking and elimination. This means that pigs who are active (move, eat, drink or manipulate enrichment) do not disturb sleeping pigs, or enrichment does not get soiled with manure. Sleeping areas should be avoided. Resting (but not sleeping) pigs often explore the floor. This means that substrate racks can be placed near the edge of resting areas.

It is helpful to install permanent attachment devices (for example, a T-bar between two pens, or substrate rack in the corner of two pens), so that the same location is always used. Refilling or renewing enrichment from the path in front of a pen allows easy maintenance (Figure 4.5). By observing the behaviour and vocalizations (aggression, squeals) of the pigs, you can check if the location is correct.

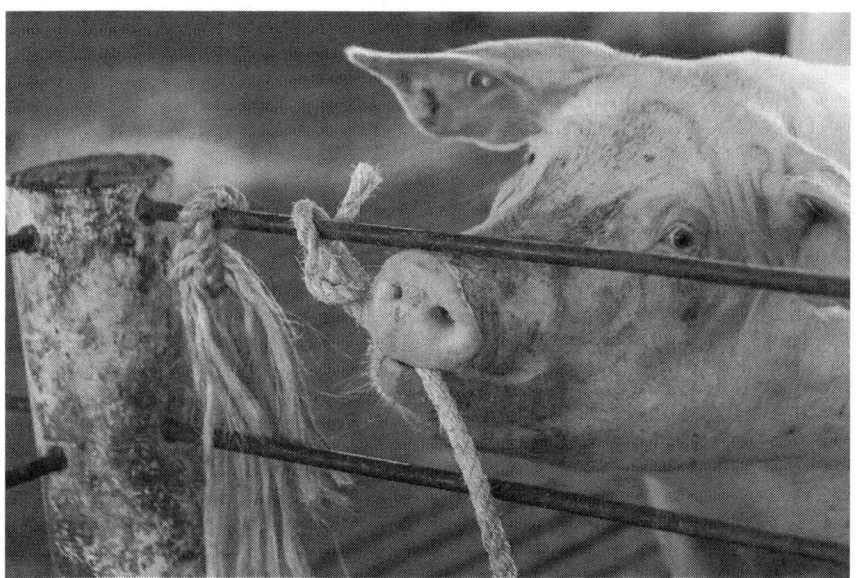

Figure 4.5 Rope to chew on. Photo: World Animal Protection/N. Castro.

4.2.6 Emergency enrichment for tail biting outbreaks

Enrichment is an important tool with which to manage tail biting, especially when the early signs of tail biting are observed (Chapter 3). Extra or different enrichment material, which is not part of the daily rotation, should be provided to ensure novelty. Objects such as salt and mineral lick stones and extra fibre can be useful to address underlying nutritional issues. It should be noted that tail biting is a multifactorial issue. Enrichment should be just one of measures taken to manage it.

TIP 3

Have emergency enrichment materials readily available at the farm so that they can be applied directly when the first signs of tail biting occur.

4.2.7 Costs

The main factors that influence the cost of providing enrichment are:

- the type of enrichment (substrate bedding, substrates in racks or point source objects)
- the renewal rate (substrates topped up daily, objects renewed regularly)
- the maintenance time (to maintain, clean and renew enrichment, including the ease of maintenance)
- whether they are commercially available or made from freely available farm materials.

Costs can be kept to a minimum by combining good quality items (such as food balls) which can be cleaned and reused with items of little or no cost, such as freshly cut branches, ice blocks or empty (paper) feed sacks.

For rearing pigs with intact tails it was calculated in 2016 that the cost of using straw was equal to 0.25% of costs in fattening farms, and from

2.8 to 4% of all costs in breeding units. (Source: EU folder 'Cutting the need for tail-docking').

4.2.8 Measure your success

In order to quantify the benefits of enrichment, it is important to monitor the long-term effects of the strategy used on farm and not only focus on the short term. Good record keeping will show the costs and benefits (Chapter 2) of an enrichment programme, and can be used to adjust management to optimize benefits.

The benefits of enrichment include:

1. prevention or reduction of damaging behaviour, such as ear and tail biting, or shorter and less severe outbreaks when managed with extra enrichment

2. calmer, more content pigs, associated with better welfare and a higher overall health

3. improved meat pig performance, resulting in reduced feed costs

4. improved sow performance (for example, lower lameness levels, lower stress levels and stereotypies, improved pregnancies, ease of farrowing, shorter partus, increased maternal care), resulting in more pigs per sow per year

5. improved (young) piglet survival (for example, coping with and adapting to weaning, reducing the growth check after weaning).

4.3 Piglet welfare

4.3.1 Large litters and pre-weaning mortality

LENE JUUL PEDERSEN AND CECILIE KOBEK-KJELDAGER

Since the beginning of the 1990s, the average litter size of production sows has been increased substantially through genetic selection. It is now common to see litter sizes in which the piglets outnumber functional teats. The most prolific genotypes give birth to an average of 17–18 live-born piglets and close to 20 total born across parities, while most sows in average have approximately 14 teats. There are economic benefits of producing large litters in terms of more weaned pigs per sow. However, it comes with a cost in terms of reduced sow and piglets welfare, and higher risks of neonatal piglet mortality.

Piglets born in large litters are smaller due to competition in the uterus for resources. Small piglets are more vulnerable to most risk factors for death, such as cold stress, starvation, crushing and disease. Therefore, large litter size is commonly related to high mortality rates. Alternative production systems, in which sows are kept loose, for example, outdoor production, seem particularly vulnerable to the negative impact of large litter sizes and may benefit more from using less prolific genotypes.

A large litter size constitutes a risk for prolonged farrowing that may put the sow at risk of dystocia and farrowing related diseases. Prolonged farrowing increases the risk of stillbirth. Live-born piglets can suffer from hypoxia during a long parturition, which may influence their brain, learning capacity and behavioural development. Such piglets have an increased risk of dying later in life. To reduce the risk of mortality and welfare problems related to, for example, crushing and starvation it is essential to have high-skilled management input during farrowing and lactation.

Birth surveillance and assistance can reduce the risk of dystocia, still-birth and early death. It may even prevent sow culling. Different surveys indicate that a considerable proportion of culled sows suffered from farrowing related problems.

Special care needs to be given to small piglets in large litters during the very first hours of life to reduce hypothermia (Figure 4.6). Research has shown that drying and warming piglets at birth reduces the risk of death. This can be done manually during supervision of the farrowing. It can also be done by heating the birth site with, for example, radiant

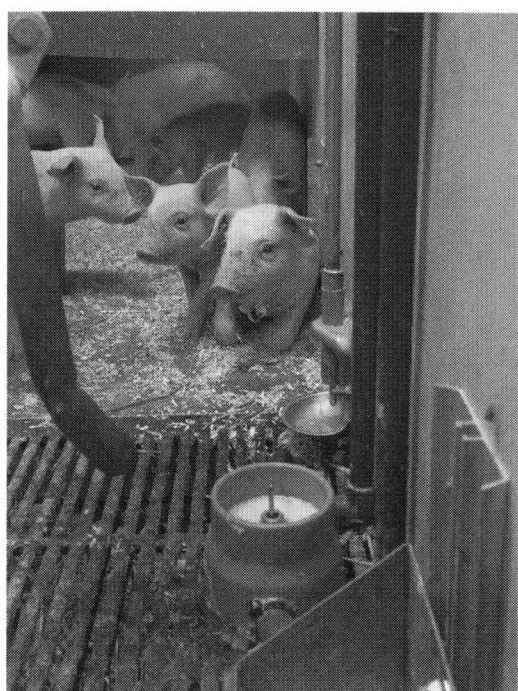

Figure 4.6 A heat lamp and extra milk to help the many piglets. Photo: Cecilie Kobek-Kjeldager.

heat or by floor heating. A similar effect can be achieved by supplying abundant straw at the birth site to dry and warm the piglet or by keeping the room temperature around 24–25°C. The last may, however, be a threat to sow welfare due to the associated risk of heat stress, and should therefore be limited to a short period around farrowing.

Pigs born in large litters get less colostrum per pig since the volume of colostrum available does not increase with litter size. Colostrum is an important supply of energy for new born pigs and their only source of immunoglobulins to protect them against diseases during the first 3–4 weeks of life. To provide colostrum to all piglets, so called 'split-suckling' can be used where the first half of a litter can be locked up in the creep area after they have had colostrum while the second half suckle colostrum. Smaller pigs can also be fed a milk replacer at birth with a syringe to ensure sufficient energy supply to initiate suckling.

Management strategies for nursing surplus piglets

Twelve to 24 hours after birth, sow colostrum gradually changes from being available continuously into a cyclic pattern. During the same period, the immunoglobulin content of colostrum is dramatically reduced. Pigs accordingly change from continuous suckling to suckling every 45–60 minutes in short bouts of 15–20 seconds where milk is available. During the short bouts of milk release all pigs need to be present with a teat in their mouth to be able to ingest milk. Pigs therefore defend a preferred teat from which they suckle during each milk let down. If there are more pigs in a litter than functional teats, some pigs lose access to a teat after a period of intensive fighting with littermates. These fights constitute a welfare threat due to social stress and increased risk of lesions on the snout and limbs. Pigs that permanently lose ownership to a teat will eventually starve to death, if not crushed beforehand. It is therefore necessary to adopt strategies to provide milk to surplus piglets of highly prolific genotypes in order to avoid severe welfare problems.

Strategies used include creating nurse sows, using Rescue Deck® and the provision of milk replacer in drinking cups or troughs outside or inside the farrowing pen.

A nurse sow, after weaning her own litter, fosters surplus new born piglets from foreign litters given to her either when she is 21 days post-partum (one-step strategy) or 7 days post-partum (two-step strategy). In the latter (two-step strategy) the nurse sow's approximately 7 days old pigs are fostered to an interim sow who is 21 days post-partum. The pigs of the interim sow are weaned. The associated welfare problems with such strategies include the risk of lesions and reduced pig growth (likely caused by pigs fighting over teats when mixed and moved, and by a declining milk supply as lactation progresses). Increased incidence of lesions on the limbs and udders of nurse sows have also been observed and the prolonged stay in a farrowing crate with a large litter compromises sow welfare.

Surplus pigs can also be taken away from the sow at birth and fostered in a Rescue Deck®. In a Rescue Deck® piglets are provided with milk replacer from drinking cups or artificial teats. This management tool results in the piglets developing abnormal behaviour, and depending on the quality of the milk replacer and pen design, it may also reduce growth. Not all member states permit Rescue Deck® use under EU welfare legislation because pigs are weaned from the sow at birth. An alternative strategy used is to provide the milk replacer inside the farrowing pen as a supplement feed source for surplus piglets. This strategy also seems to result in instability of the teat order, resulting in piglets fighting for access to teats, and reduced growth – again dependent on the quality of the milk replacer and the way it is provided.

Piglets born in large litters may – due to their smaller individual birth weight – have a poorer growth rate and thus a lower weaning weight. They may therefore also be more vulnerable to early weaning stress. A consequence may be reduced post-weaning growth, higher risk of weaning diarrhoea and increased need for antibiotics. Behavioural problems, such as belly nosing and tail and ear biting, may also be related to the pre-weaning stress caused by the increased competition. However, the prolonged negative effects of the pre-weaning environment require further research.

Increasing the number of weaned piglets using prolific sows can be economically viable up to a certain limit. When the average number of born piglets, however, outnumber the available teats then the cost of keeping surplus piglets alive is likely to increase dramatically. The costs are not only in increased labour, but also in terms of reduced growth and poor animal welfare. The continued increase in litter size may also raise ethical concerns.

4.3.2 Management procedures

SARAH ISON

Pigs have similar anatomical structures and bodily functions as humans; if something would be painful to us, it is painful to a pig. Pigs express pain with behaviour, vocalizations, facial expression and substances in blood or other bodily fluids. Production indicators, such as growth, can be an indirect sign, as pain can reduce feed and water intake. The recognition of pain indicators has come through studying piglets undergoing management procedures: castration, tail docking, teeth reduction, ear notching/tagging and injections (for example, iron). Careful observation is needed as piglets may hide pain from potential predators, including well-meaning stockpeople. Painful early life experiences also have longer-term negative impacts for pigs as they do in humans.

Welfare can be improved by changing piglet management routines, such as adopting the the 3Rs approach: reduction (fewer pigs undergoing procedures); replacement (using alternatives techniques); or refinement (providing anaesthetic and/or pain relief). Ideal solutions are those that replace painful procedures; both saving time on piglet processing and offering other welfare, production or meat quality benefits. For instance, injections can be replaced with orally administered products or needleless injectors that avoid damaging muscle tissue.

Tail docking (Section 4.4.2) and teeth reduction mask other issues and can feasibly be replaced in many situations. Alternatives to teeth reduction involve managing large litters (Section 4.3.1), ensuring sow health and sow comfort (including lying comfort), and only considering teeth reduction as a last resort when other management action fails to reduce face or udder damage.

Castration is an invasive procedure involving skin, deep tissue and organs resulting in moderate to severe pain. Castration reduces unwanted sexual and aggressive behaviour and 'boar taint', an unpleasant odour in pork associated with substances (androstenone, skatole and indole) that increases in boars from puberty. Physical castration can be replaced by raising boars with careful management to reduce the impacts of sexual and/or aggressive behaviour and boar taint detection on the slaughter line. The use of anaesthetic and pain relief to refine castration has been studied, but pain during and after the procedure cannot be convincingly reduced to an acceptable level on a commercial scale with the drugs approved to treat food-producing animals. Alternatively, immunocastration involves two or three injections stimulating the pig's immune system, like a vaccine, to block the build-up of substances leading to boar taint and reducing problem behaviour. Marketing boars or immunocastrated barrows has economic advantages from improved growth, feed efficiency and meat quality attributes.

4.3.3 Euthanasia

MONIQUE D. PAIRIS-GARCIA

As mentioned earlier in this chapter, for some piglets survival or recovery is extremely unlikely regardless of the supportive care provided on farm. In these situations, it is our ethical obligation as farmers, veterinarians and animal caretakers to end the suffering of that animal by performing timely euthanasia with an approved method. Timely euthanasia should be implemented when the likelihood of recovery is poor and the animal is experiencing pain and suffering. Timely euthanasia reflects compassion of the caretaker and should never be viewed as a failure.

Currently, there are several euthanasia options that can be performed on neonatal piglets. Manual blunt force trauma has been shown to result in immediate unconsciousness and rapid death when performed correctly. According to the National Pork Board On-Farm Euthanasia of Swine Recommendations, blunt force trauma is effective in pigs less than 5.5 kg (12 lbs) and is conducted by applying a quick, firm blow to the top of the head over the brain, as illustrated in Figure 4.7. This method, however, is not aesthetically pleasing to the general public and some caretakers are not comfortable performing this technique.

Alternative techniques approved by the American Veterinary Medical Association for neonatal piglet euthanasia include gas euthanasia and non-penetrating captive bolt gun. Gas euthanasia results in loss of

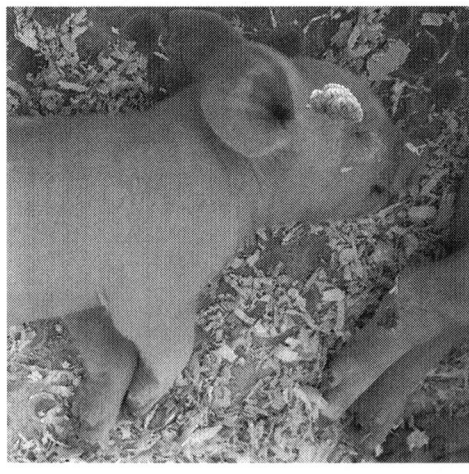

Figure 4.7 Pigs' brains are small and surrounded by a thick skull. The blow in manual blunt force trauma should be firm and exact on the location indicated. Photo: J.R. Yee.

consciousness immediately followed by death. Commercially available carbon dioxide euthanasia systems are available that allow caretakers to euthanize piglets in a humane and consistent manner on farm at an investment of approximately €2600.

Non-penetrating captive bolt guns work in the same manner as blunt force trauma but the piglet remains stationary. Consistency and efficacy are often improved when using this more controlled method. Several non-penetrating captive bolt guns have come out in the market in the past years. Some of the guns allow for use of the captive bolt gun for piglets (non-penetrating head) as well as for sows and boars (penetrating head). Non-penetrating captive bolt guns powered by a standard air compressor (120 psi) can euthanize piglets up to 9 kg. This also allows caretakers to easily conduct a second shot if needed and it can be utilized around the farm by attaching the gun to a transportable compressed-gas canister. For more details on non-penetrative captive bolt guns see the article by Grist et al. (2018).

Euthanasia is a sensitive and emotive topic for both the public and those directly caring for piglets. It is imperative that we humanely euthanize compromised piglets in a timely manner to minimize pain and distress and to recognize that the quality of the animal's death is as important a welfare concern as the quality of its life.

Reference

Grist, A., Lines, J., Knowles, T., Mason, C. and Wotton, S. (2018). The Use of a Non-Penetrating Captive Bolt for the Euthanasia of Neonate Piglets. *Animals*, *8*(4), p.48.

4.4 Welfare from weaning to fattening

4.4.1 Weaning

JOHN J. MCGLONE

Weaning refers to stopping nursing or suckling by piglets, usually by separating sows and piglets. Among wild pigs, weaning can happen naturally by a gradual process over a period of weeks. Wild or feral pigs will wean their piglets slowly when they are a few months old. On commercial farms, piglets are removed from their sow during weaning. The sow often returns to the breeding herd and the piglets go to a post-weaning nursery barn, pen or pasture. Abrupt weaning is clearly stressful to both the sow and the piglets.

Weaning age has decreased on commercial farms over the past 100 years. Economics drove the decrease in weaning age. If sows are weaned earlier, they will have more pigs per sow per year. For example, if weaning age decreases from 8 weeks to 4 weeks of age, the cycle from breeding to weaning is reduced by 4 weeks. With 8-week weaning, the cycle of gestation plus lactation is 170 days (114 + 56 days) and one would have 2.1 litters per sow per year. If pigs are weaned at 4 weeks of age, the gestation plus lactation cycle is 142 days and one would have 2.6 litters per sow per year. If sows average 10 pigs weaned, 8-week weaning would produce 21 pigs per sow per year while 4-week weaning would produce 26 pigs per sow per year. Getting those extra pigs with the same sow herd is economically advantageous and improves the sustainability of pork production. The sow herd has a certain footprint in terms of environmental impact, labour costs and cost to maintain the adult females. If those sows produce more pigs on the same footprint, this has many advantages. But the earlier pigs are weaned, the more behavioural problems emerge among both sows and piglets.

Pigs and sows were weaned at 8 weeks of age 50 to 100+ years ago. In the 1960s, commercial farms began what was then called early weaning at 4 weeks of age. Then, economics drove weaning age to 21 days. People found value in even earlier weaning in terms of improving piglet health. Today, in North America, the most common weaning age is 17–23 days while in parts of Europe, weaning age is 28 days or later. Some farmers use segregated early weaning (SEW) to reduce disease transmission. SEW piglets are weaned from 5 to 20 days of age.

The sow experiences stress after weaning. Her stress is manifest in two areas: (1) her anatomy and physiology and (2) her behaviour. Abrupt piglet removal causes each sow's udder to swell with milk that is not being suckled. The udder gets hot and uncomfortable. Sow feed intake drops rapidly. Weaned sows become less active, lethargic and perhaps depressed. Within a week, the weaned sow is typically bred and by that point, her udder and general behaviour are improved. Little can be done to relieve this physical and psychological stress among weaned sows. And because this short-term sow stress has little economic cost, little research is directed at trying to reduce this stress in weaned sows.

Piglets have a much greater stress response at weaning. Piglets have multiple problems in the post-weaning environment, including physical, thermal, nutritional and psychological issues. Piglets have a less-than-fully developed immune system and gastrointestinal tract (stomach and intestines). If they experience a stressor at this immature state, they are more likely to have digestive or respiratory illness.

Piglets must be kept warm since they do not have the sow to lie against. If these young pigs get chilled, they are more likely to get sick. Studies have shown that microbial diseases (bacteria and virus) that do not make a 6-month old pig sick, can easily make a weaned pig ill if they are chilled.

Piglets experience an abrupt change of diet. Piglets consume mostly milk up to 3 weeks of age, even if they are offered dry food during lactation. When they are placed in a post-weaning nursery environment, they will not eat for 12 to 24 hours. The dry diet may contain grain, soybean meal, vitamins, minerals and even a little dry milk. This dry food is a lower plane of nutrition than natural sow milk. Piglets typically lose body weight the first few days after weaning, then they begin to gradually eat and grow again. Piglets may be the same weight 1 week after weaning as they were at weaning. Then, they will start growing at an increasingly rapid rate.

Piglets are also abruptly removed from their mother's odours. Compared to feral pigs, both adult male and adult female odours are missing in the post-weaning environment. Restoration of the maternal odours in the post-weaning environment has been shown in university trials to reduce the stress of weaning. Maternal odours (called pheromones) are gradually adopted by commercial farms. The nursery environment is deficient in adult odours and this causes problems for the piglets in the same way that missing a nutrient in their diet would cause problems. This is an area in which improvements in pig performance and welfare will be found in the future.

Piglets also spend a significant amount of time fighting because piglets from different litters are often kept in the same pens. In the wild, piglets from other sows are interacting with each other continually. Because lactating litters are often housed in single-litter pens or crates, they do not develop social skills in a healthy manner. Like most species, when novel animals are encountered, fights can begin. Piglet fighting causes weight loss and injury (Section 4.4.3). When enrichment is provided, such as ropes (Figure 4.8), pigs often fight less. Enrichment may reduce other behavioural problems as well.

Piglets sometimes show what is called abnormal or aberrant behaviours. These include navel sucking, ear biting, tail biting, and belly or side rubbing. These abnormal behaviours increase with early weaning, which

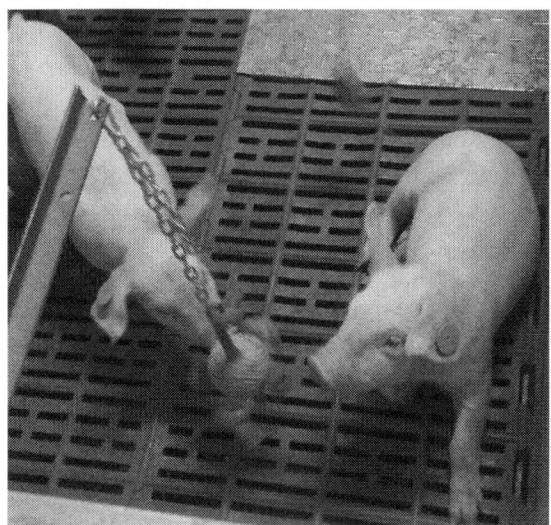

Figure 4.8
Providing environmental enrichment can reduce post-weaning aggressive behaviour. Photo: I. Camerlink.

suggests they are expressed because of a lack of suckling at an age in which they are biologically programmed to suckle (3 to 10 weeks of age). Other environmental stressors, such as high ammonia, dust, infectious disease or limited food or water, will increase the rate of abnormal behaviours.

The best practices for weaned pigs include providing a warm, draft-free pen with ample space. If piglets experience clean air and a comfortable environment, they will have less long-term problems with their growth, health and behaviour. Enrichments can include meaningful physical toys or objects to interact with and comforting smells that can reduce stress in the weaned pigs.

4.4.2 Tail biting

ANNA VALROS

A curly, intact tail is a classical sign of a healthy pig (Figure 4.9). However, tail biting is a regrettably common and challenging, damaging behaviour

Figure 4.9 A curly, intact tail, and a shortened, but healed tail. Photo: A. Valros.

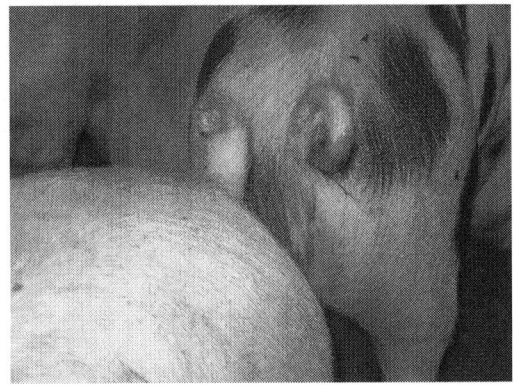

in pigs in modern production. Tail biting lesions cause pain and stress, and an increased risk of infections. Tail lesions also decrease the economic result, through increased medication costs, increased workload, carcass losses and mortality. However, it is crucial to remember that tail biting in itself is a sign of reduced welfare, and any measures to reduce the behaviour will also increase the welfare of the pig. Thus, tail docking, which decreases the prevalence of tail lesions, does not fix the underlying problem, nor abolish the behaviour itself. In countries, such as Finland, where tail docking is totally banned, producers tend to use the tail as a measure of success – a pen with curly tailed pigs indicates that management is appropriate. Thus, the state of the tail is a good iceberg indicator for good husbandry practice.

Why do pigs bite tails?

Even though the exact motivation for tail biting remains a mystery, it is well established that tail biting is related to a reduced welfare. Thus, anything that potentially cause pigs stress, frustration or other types of negative states is a risk factor for tail biting. Several types of tail biting have been suggested by research, and the motivation behind these might differ.

1. Two-stage tail biting usually results in mild or moderate tail lesions in several pigs, often in several pens. Two-stage tail biting escalates from non-damaging manipulation of other pigs' tails to damaging biting, possibly caused by frustration due to some chronic problem in the piggery, such a lack of manipulable materials. Thus, if this type of biting occurs regularly, management should be modified to better meet the needs of the pig, such as allowing for appropriate exploration of the environment.

2. If pigs encounter competition for resources, such as feed, they might revert to sudden-forceful tail biting to gain access to the resource. In these cases, severely bitten tails might occur very suddenly in only one or a few pigs. If so, one should consider adding feeding space, water nipples, or other resources that are crucial for the pigs' well-being.

3. In some cases, producers can clearly identify the biter, either as the only unbitten pig in a pen, or as a pig continuously biting other pigs. Such obsessive biters are often anecdotally described as having a 'mad glare' in their eyes. These pigs have probably encountered severe challenges at some point of their lives, and have taken on biting tails as a coping strategy. They should be removed from the pen to avoid further damage. If this is reoccurring on the farm, there is a need to check for risk factors that might cause some pigs to suffer from severe stress during rearing.

4. Maybe the most feared type of tail biting is one that suddenly spreads like an epidemic. Everything is fine in the evening, but next morning lots of tails have been severely bitten. This is typically caused by sudden changes: such as feeder malfunction, temperature increase or ventilation failure, causing a decrease in air quality. Owing to the unpredictable nature of this type of tail biting, it is difficult to totally avoid, but by ensuring proper function of technology and installing alarm systems, the risks can be reduced.

How can the tail biting risk be reduced on-farm?

As mentioned above, tail biting behaviour might have different motivational backgrounds. Identifying these is a first step towards solving problems on a specific farm.

Especially in cases where tail biting is a reoccurring problem, or if a farm that is currently docking wants to move towards rearing intact-tailed pigs, there is a need to make a holistic risk assessment. Tail biting is a multifactorial problem, with risk factors adding up to increase the risk, and there are usually no quick-fix solutions. The more risk factors that can be corrected, the better. Typical chronic risk factors include poor environment, such as poor ventilation, inappropriate temperature and poor pen design. Another set of risk factors is competition for resources, such as food, water and preferred resting places. A high disease pressure, and nutritional deficiencies or poor water availability further increase the risk for tail biting. One of the most commonly mentioned risk factors is inadequate use of proper manipulable material. Chains, plastic tubes and other point-source objects might be good additions to pens, but the pigs should be given material that is among other characteristics chewable, rootable and easily accessible (see Section 4.2 for the key characteristics of suitable enrichment for the various age categories). Good alternatives include straw, hay or peat, paper, cardboard and ropes of natural materials. For more information on appropriate enrichment, see Section 4.2.

Particularly when tail biting only occurs as sporadic epidemics, it is important to also reduce the risk of suddenly occurring negative changes in the pigs' environment ('acute' risk factors). Examples of such measures were given earlier. However, as tail biting is caused by the additive effect of a large number of risk factors, the better the chronic risk factors mentioned above are managed, the lower is the risk that acute ones cause an outbreak.

Early detection and intervention

Even on a farm where both chronic and acute risk factors have been minimized, there is a certain risk of outbreaks occurring occasionally. As outbreaks can be difficult to stop when they have escalated, early detection of upcoming outbreaks is of utmost importance. When the first wounded tail is noticed, the outbreak is already ongoing. Typical signs of an upcoming outbreak include increases in activity, restlessness, changes in feeding or drinking patterns and specifically, hanging tails, or tails tucked between the legs, as described in Section 3.1.2 on tail posture (Figure 4.10). As soon as any of these changes are noticed, action should be taken. Automatic early warning systems for hanging tails are being developed. There should be a readily available 'first aid kit' (see also Section 4.6) on each farm, including manipulable materials of high interest to the pigs, and which are totally novel to the specific group of pigs. If adding these is not enough, the biter should be removed from the pen. Also severely bitten pigs can be removed to a hospital pen, and should be treated appropriately.

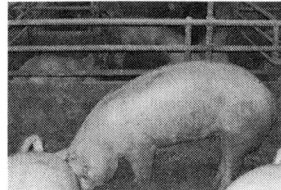 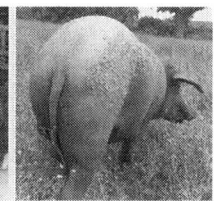

Figure 4.10 Pigs with tucked tails calls for immediate attention. Photo: A. Valros, I. Camerlink.

How to reach the goal?

Figure 4.11 illustrates the components of a farm-specific action plan for systematically reducing the occurrence of tail biting lesions. In some countries, farmers get regular feedback from the slaughterhouse on the percentage of tail lesions in each batch of pigs. The occurrence of tail lesions should, however, be assessed also at the farm level to allow for a follow-up of how well the farm-specific action plan is working, and to identify production stages and seasons where the risk for tail biting is highest, and thus, when there is a need for special attention to the pigs.

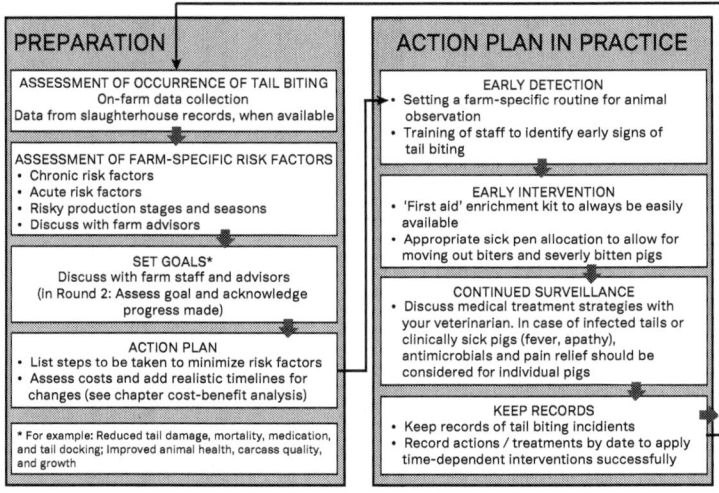

PREPARATION

ASSESSMENT OF OCCURRENCE OF TAIL BITING
On-farm data collection
Data from slaughterhouse records, when available

ASSESSMENT OF FARM-SPECIFIC RISK FACTORS
• Chronic risk factors
• Acute risk factors
• Risky production stages and seasons
• Discuss with farm advisors

SET GOALS*
Discuss with farm staff and advisors
(In Round 2: Assess goal and acknowledge progress made)

ACTION PLAN
• List steps to be taken to minimize risk factors
• Assess costs and add realistic timelines for changes (see chapter cost-benefit analysis)

* For example: Reduced tail damage, mortality, medication, and tail docking; improved animal health, carcass quality, and growth

ACTION PLAN IN PRACTICE

EARLY DETECTION
• Setting a farm-specific routine for animal observation
• Training of staff to identify early signs of tail biting

EARLY INTERVENTION
• 'First aid' enrichment kit to always be easily available
• Appropriate sick pen allocation to allow for moving out biters and severely bitten pigs

CONTINUED SURVEILLANCE
• Discuss medical treatment strategies with your veterinarian. In case of infected tails or clinically sick pigs (fever, apathy), antimicrobials and pain relief should be considered for individual pigs

KEEP RECORDS
• Keep records of tail biting incidents
• Record actions / treatments by date to apply time-dependent interventions successfully

Figure 4.11 Action plan to reduce tail biting. Illustration: A. Valros.

4.4.3 Aggression

SIMON P. TURNER

Unfamiliar pigs are motivated to establish dominance relationships. Pigs of similar weight or with aggressive personalities will use damaging fighting to do this. This behaviour is very different in motivation from tail biting (Section 4.4.2). Fighting can lead to many skin lesions (scratches) particularly around the neck and shoulders, as shown in Figure 4.12. Fighting can depress growth and immunity and increase the risk of lameness.

Research has shown that the use of sedatives or mixing pigs at night or in low light levels tends to delay but not reduce fighting. None of these strategies remove the motivation to fight. Depending on the country, some of these strategies may also contravene legislation.

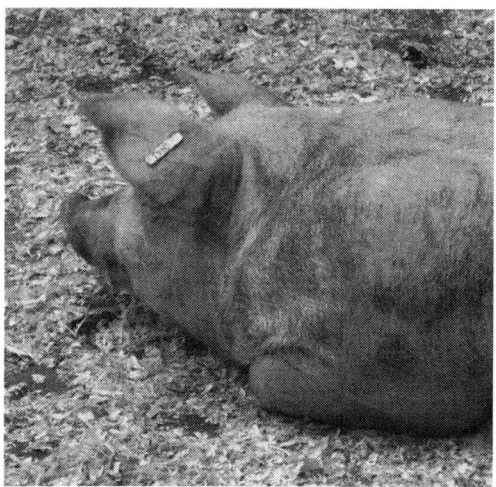

Figure 4.12 Skin lesions on the shoulder after fighting. Photo: SRUC / M. Farish.

Fighting is best reduced by avoiding mixing unfamiliar pigs. If planning a new building, try to ensure that it complements the group sizes used in existing buildings to avoid mixing between growth stages.

Try to mix pigs as young as possible as they then fight less severely. Many producers now mix pigs into large groups at weaning and reduce the group size without mixing as they move into later growth stages.

The best strategies to reduce fighting help pigs establish dominance relationships quickly and efficiently. The best ways to achieve this are as follows.

1. Let pigs meet before weaning. Research is unanimous that allowing adjacent litters of piglets to mix at around 2 weeks of age reduces fighting when these pigs meet new animals at weaning (Figure 4.13). No growth penalty is seen when the litters are of similar weight. This benefit continues beyond the grower stage.

2. Give pigs space to signal defeat. Prolonged bullying of the loser by the winner occurs if the loser does not have the space to properly signal defeat.

3. Use large group sizes at weaning. At very large group sizes (>100 pigs) the amount of injuries per pig is slightly reduced.

4. Give them somewhere to hide. Provide an obstacle behind which pigs can hide; some research suggests that this reduces injuries.

Once dominance relationships are established they must be maintained. If large numbers of new injuries are present in well established groups the likely cause is competition for access to feed, water or a dry comfortable lying area. Competition will cause subordinate pigs to challenge dominant ones leading to ongoing aggression.

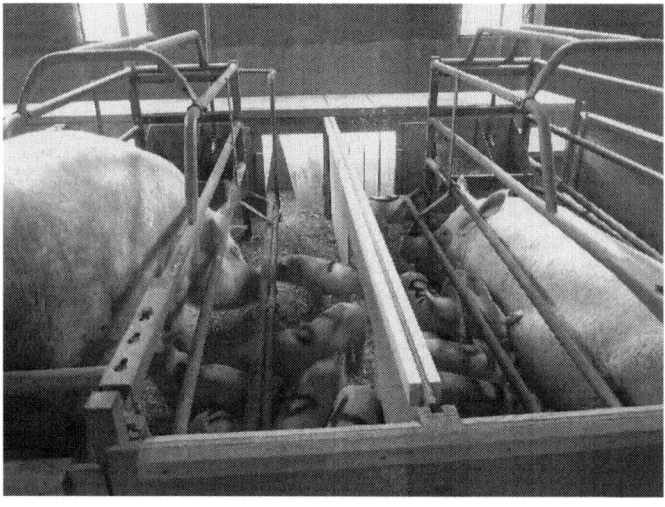

Figure 4.13 Socialization of piglets by joining two litters together. Photo: SRUC / M. Farish.

4.5 Welfare of boars

LOTTA RYDHMER

Male piglets have been surgically castrated through history, all over the world. In ancient times pigs were castrated to increase fat content and facilitate management. Today the main reason is to avoid boar taint in meat. There is, however, a consensus within the EU: that painful surgical castration should be avoided.

Although entire male pigs are spared from pain during and after surgery there are other welfare issues associated with their rearing. Aggression is more common among entire males than among castrates. Sexual behaviour also causes welfare problems. Thus entire male pigs need to be handled with great care.

Entire male pigs grow faster, use feed more efficiently and are leaner and more muscled at slaughter, compared to castrates and females. The sex hormone testosterone is synthesized in the testes. Raised levels of testosterone and other hormones at puberty are usually associated with more sexual and aggressive behaviours, such as fighting, head-knocking, threatening and biting. Most pigs fight when they meet unfamiliar pigs, but entire males fight more. A higher level of the boar pheromone androstenone is also associated with more aggressive behaviour.

In general, pigs in a stable group become less active and less aggressive with increasing age. There is, however, a variation between individuals and aggressive individuals continue to show more aggressive behaviour than others over time. Not all pigs attack others, but any pig may become a victim. In sex-mixed pens, entire males show more aggressive behaviour than females, but entire males and females receive equal amounts of aggression.

Fast-growing pigs are more aggressive than slow-growing pigs and within a pen the heaviest pigs are usually the most aggressive ones. They are also the ones that eat first if there is a competition at feeding. If these fast-growing pigs are sent to slaughter before the rest, the level of aggression among the remaining pigs in the pen does, however, not always decrease. It may even increase when the pigs have to establish a new hierarchy.

Entire males perform more sexual behaviour (mounts and attempts to mount) than castrates and females (Figure 4.14), which causes skin lesions on pen mates. A high frequency of penile injuries has also been observed. If female pigs are present in the pen they get mated and some become pregnant. Slaughter of pregnant pigs should be questioned on ethical grounds. With lots of mounting and aggression in the pen, the risk of leg problems increases. In pens where entire males and females are mixed, pigs of both sexes are mounted equally often. Some pigs

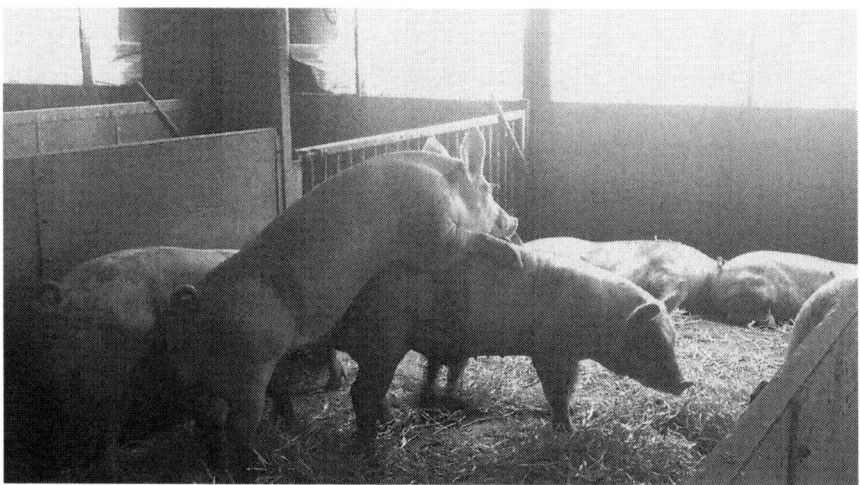

Figure 4.14 Mounting behaviour in boars. Photo: I. Camerlink.

in the pen are, however, not involved at all and they have less skin lesions. Entire males that do not mount, grow faster than entire males mounting other pigs.

Pigs are social animals and entire males perform more social interactions, such as sniffing, pushing and manipulating ears and tails than castrates. In some studies, entire males seem to be more active; they have less time for resting. Furthermore, entire males are dirtier than castrates and female pigs, and the pen hygiene is lower when there are entire males.

Pigs are often sent to slaughter at a certain weight and since there is a variation in growth rate all pigs in a pen are not slaughtered at the same time. It is common practice to mix pigs from different pens on the truck and at the slaughterhouse. Mixing unfamiliar entire males prior to slaughter provokes lots of aggressive behaviour and mounting. This leads to a high frequency of skin lesions, which can be seen on the carcasses and may also reduce meat quality.

With a higher risk of boar taint in addition to all the welfare issues presented above – is there any reason to rear entire males instead of castrates? There must be, since castration of pigs is uncommon in some countries, for example, in the UK. In fact, there are at least two strong arguments against castration.

1. Surgical castration leads to reduced feed efficiency and increased environmental impact due to higher fat deposition among castrated pigs, compared to entire males.

2. Surgical castration leads to reduced welfare due to the pain, fear and distress that piglets experience during and shortly after castration.

As in the beginning of this chapter, surgical castration of pigs should be avoided. Immunocastration is a good alternative to surgical castration from a welfare perspective, but immunocastrated males are less efficient (slower growth and reduced feed efficiency) than entire males.

A sustainable pig production includes environmental, economic and social aspects, and animal welfare is one of these social aspects. How should entire male pigs be handled, in order to decrease the risk of welfare problems?

TIPS

1. The first recommendation is to separate males and females at weaning. In this way, at least half of all pigs are spared from mountings and aggressions from the entire males. Rearing male and female pigs in separate pens also gives the possibility to fully use the higher growth potential of entire males by using different feeding regimes.

2. The second recommendation is to avoid disturbances and strive for a calm rearing environment. Entire male pigs are more reactive than castrates and a disturbance like regrouping provokes aggression and triggers mounting. Feeding wet feed in a long trough reduces competition and thereby aggressive interactions and skin lesions.

3. The third recommendation is to send all entire males from the same pen to slaughter at the same time without mixing them with other pigs on the truck or at the slaughterhouse. This may require changes in the design of trucks and lairage pens. It also requires retailers willing to market pork with a larger variation, for example, in size of cutlets.

Taking a longer-term perspective, genetic selection against aggressive behaviour would improve welfare. The trait is heritable, but time consuming to record. New recording techniques based on sensors or image analysis may open up for more practical recording solutions, and non-aggressive behaviour may be a selection trait in the future. Selection against sexual behaviour is, however, more problematic; sexual behaviour is part of reproduction and high reproduction is an important breeding goal trait.

Ideally, entire males shall be reared in intact litter groups to increase their welfare. However, housing males from only one litter in each pen until slaughter would result in very small groups and thus increase rearing costs. There is one period in life when unknown pigs can meet without fighting; when they are 10–14 days old. At that time, piglets can be socialized by opening up between adjacent farrowing pens (see also Section 4.4.3). At weaning, such a group of several litters can be sorted by sex so that each sub-group has the right size for the growing-finishing unit. Thus, mixing with unknown pigs can be avoided. Piglet socializing and keeping intact groups during the growing-finishing phase will improve pig welfare.

4.6 Welfare of lactating sows

4.6.1 Nest building

EMMA M. BAXTER

Nest-building behaviour is a behavioural pattern typically displayed by sows 16–24 hours before they give birth (farrow), as seen in Figure 4.15. It is triggered by hormones, including an increase in prolactin. Sows perform very specific patterns of behaviour: they increase their restlessness and activity levels, carry substrate, dig and root at the ground trying to create a hollow and then manipulate and arrange the substrate to create the nest. Interacting with these environmental stimuli influences hormone levels, including an increase in oxytocin as the active nesting phase is complete 3–7 hours pre-farrowing. The sow becomes less active, lies down and goes into a 'quiet phase' before farrowing begins.

A sow will attempt to perform nest-building behaviour no matter what environment she is kept in. Sows kept in farrowing crates or pens with no nest-building material will redirect their behaviours to the pen equipment and perform bar-biting, manipulate the drinker and root and paw at the floor.

Nest building demonstrates the sow's desire to construct an environment for farrowing and lactating that can protect her offspring from predators and poor weather. A common myth is that modern domestic breeds do not nest build as they do not need to and because it has been bred out of them. This is incorrect. Despite years of domestication and selective breeding and despite protective, warm environments being

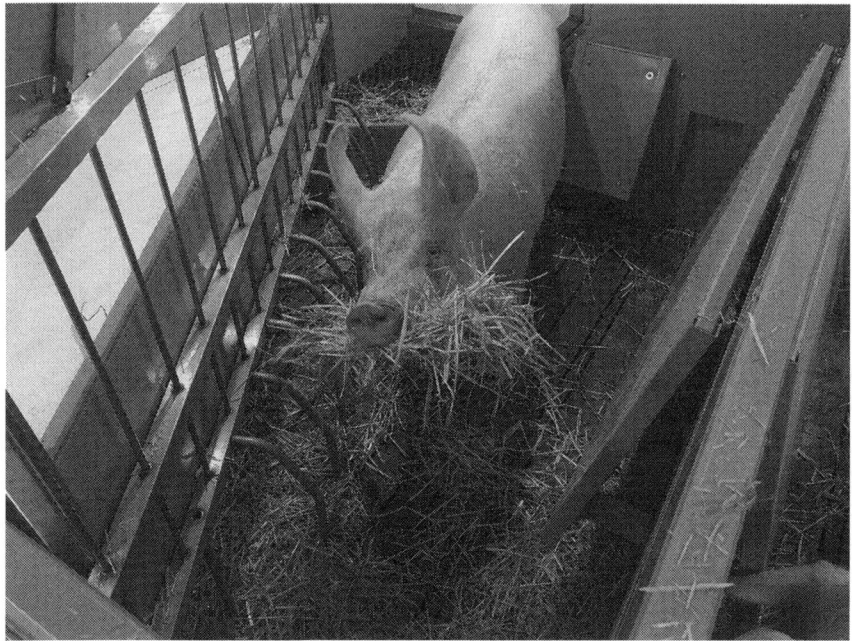

Figure 4.15 A sow collecting nest materials. Photo: SRUC / M. Farish.

provided to piglets the modern domestic sow continues to be highly motivated to nest build and perform the various behavioural patterns displayed during nest building. It is a highly motivated behavioural need and it would be counter-productive to try to breed it out of pigs, as it is considered a functional behaviour – that is, it has a purpose.

1. It influences maternal hormones.

2. It prepares the sow for farrowing.

3. It can influence her maternal behaviour.

   - Good, satisfied nest-building behaviour leads to calm farrowing behaviour and safe passage to the udder for piglets.
   - Poor, unsatisfied nest-building behaviour leads to restlessness

during farrowing, increases stress and can lead to piglet-directed aggression.

4. It can influence the success of suckling for the piglets once born.

- Piglets from mothers who have good nest-building opportunities have better immunity (higher immunoglobulin levels) because of their suckling success.

To nest build properly the sow needs certain things from her environment:

- space – to increase her activity levels and 'seek' a separate nest site and to turn around and create the nest
- substrate – to perform manipulation of nesting materials and get a sense of nest completion
- enclosure – to be able to withdraw from the herd and isolate herself and to give the nest site a sense of protection
- suitable flooring – to keep substrate in the nest.

In many countries, it is a legal requirement to provide sows with nest-building material. EU legislation (Council Directive 2008/120/EC) states that 'in the week before the expected farrowing time, sows and gilts must be given suitable nesting material in sufficient quantity unless it is not technically feasible for the slurry system used'. Even if the slurry system prevents 'sufficient quantity' of nest-building material there are ways that farmers can provide materials in the farrowing crate or on a system with fully slatted floors that would improve sow welfare and allow her to redirect her nest-building behaviour to more suitable materials.

A large quantity (at least 2 kg) of long-stemmed straw is the optimal nest-building material. Alternatives for sows on fully slatted systems include:

- hessian sacks (or jute/burlap), see also Figure 4.16
- shredded and whole paper sheets, see also Figure 4.16
- ropes made of natural fibres (not synthetic material).

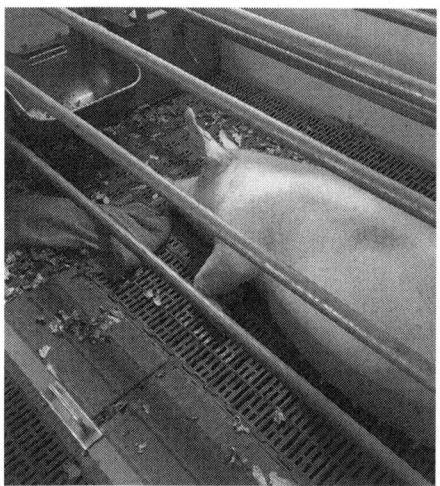

Figure 4.16 A burlap sack as alternative in slatted systems. It can also be attached to the crate. Photo: SRUC / M. Farish.

Hessian sacks and ropes must be affixed properly to prevent them falling down the slats or going behind the sow and out of her reach. For example, affix the sacks and/or rope to the side of the farrowing crate so that the sows can reach the material easily.

To fully allow satisfactory nest-building behaviour the sow requires more space, to be able to turn around and increase her activity levels. Alternative farrowing systems to the farrowing crate that do not constrain the sow would allow for this very important behaviour.

4.6.2 Farrowing

EMMA M. BAXTER

The majority of farrowing sows give birth in farrowing crates, which pose a welfare dilemma; the restriction of sow movement interferes with the performance of species-specific behaviours, such as nest building, orientation, exploration and communication with the piglets, and leads to increased physiological stress. Sows also show reduced feed and water intake and can develop pressure sores when housed in crates.

However, allowing the sow more freedom to perform motivated behaviours often results in increased crushing of piglets and hence a piglet welfare problem. Although crates are there to protect the piglets there is an increased risk of stillbirth as farrowing duration can be extended in crates. There are limited enrichment opportunities for piglets (Section 4.2).

Allowing greater freedom of movement for the sow and providing suitable substrate results in more satisfactory nest-building opportunities and a number of other welfare and performance benefits have been reported for both sows and piglets including, for sows:

- improved maternal behaviour
- improved communication with piglets
- lower stress levels for sows
- shorter farrowing durations
- reduced risk of pressure sores developing
- reduced risk of lameness
- increased feed and water intake
- improved sow metabolism.

And for piglets:

- lower risk of stillbirth
- increased suckling success (through improved oxytocin concentrations in sows and better colostrum intake and easier udder access)
- improved immune status
- higher weaning weights
- increased play behaviour leading to improved social behaviours post-weaning.

When designing farrowing systems we should ask the questions 'who are the main users of the system' and 'what are the functions that they need the system to perform?'. The primary users who interact with the system 100% of the time are the animals, the next largest users are the stockworkers.

A farrowing and lactation system should satisfy the 'Triangle of Needs' between the sow, her piglets and the stockworkers (Figure 4.17). One aspect all three 'users' want from a system is good piglet survival and any alternative must deliver piglet survival figures that are equal to or better than those reported from farrowing crates.

There are a wide variety of alternative farrowing systems that vary in how well they meet the needs of various stakeholders. Systems can be grouped within broader categories based on common features.

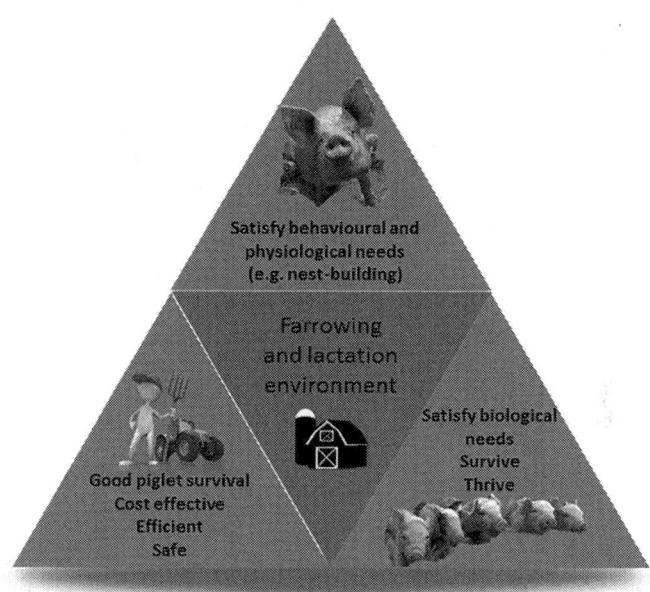

Figure 4.17 Summary of the 'triangle of need' between sows, piglets and stockworkers. Illustration: adapted from www.freefarrowing.org.

Temporary crates

The majority of temporary crates involve a widening of the existing farrowing crate to either allow the sow to be able to turn around throughout farrowing and lactation or restrain the sow during farrowing before opening the crate up approximately 5–7 days post-farrowing (Figure 4.18). These systems typically have the same footprint as a conventional farrowing crate space (approximately 4.3 m²), are built on fully slatted floors and retain the ability to restrain the sow if necessary. These systems allow loose-lactation but are not considered true free farrowing systems.

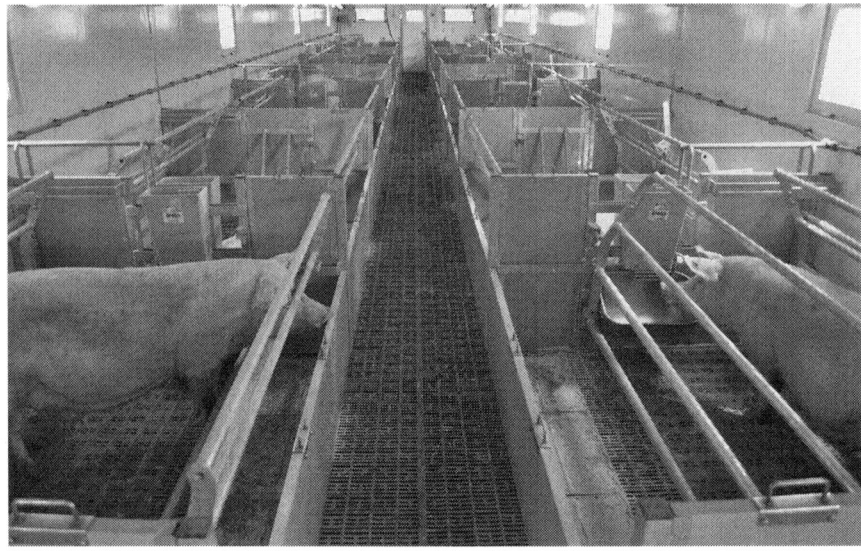

Figure 4.18 Temporary crating system. 360° Farrower in open (left side) and closed (right side) position. Photo: SRUC / M. Farish.

Zero-confinement

True free farrowing systems have no ability to confine the sow during farrowing or lactation. These include simple pens, designed pens, multi-suckle/group systems and outdoor or free range systems.

Simple pens

These systems include a range of modified designs in which the crate is absent. They attempt to occupy a similar footprint to that of the conventional farrowing crate, often with fully slatted floors, to facilitate good pen hygiene. Legislation says that 'farrowing pens where sows are kept loose must have some means of protecting the piglets, such as farrowing rails'. So simple pens often have rails around the pen walls.

Designed pens

Designed pens differ from simple pens because they have separate areas in the pen to fulfil different functions including separate dunging and lying areas, as well as additional pen 'furniture', such as rails or sloped walls, to help control the sow posture changes and protect piglets. The footprint for these sort of pens varies depending on manufacturer from 5–8.5 m² (for example PigSAFE, Figure 4.19).

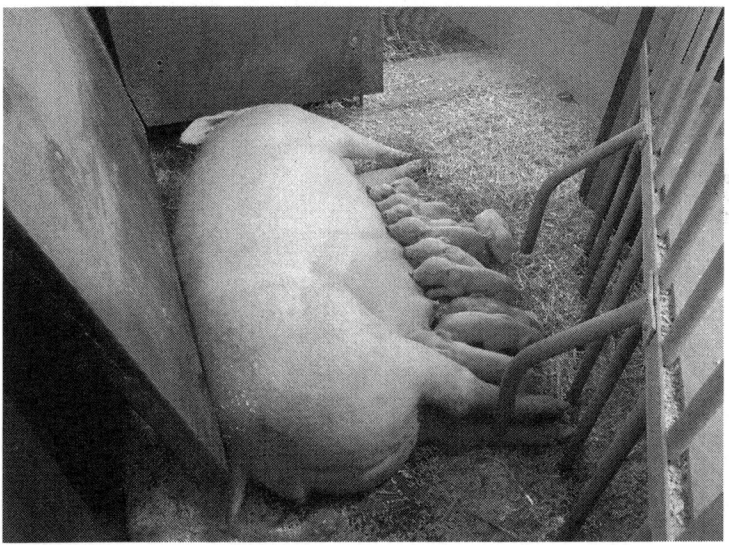

Figure 4.19 The PigSAFE pen. Photo: SRUC / M. Farish.

Group or multi-suckle systems

These systems allow sows and litters to mix before weaning. Both sows and piglets are afforded much greater space and systems are often deep-straw bedded. For farrowing, sows are initially individually housed in pens but are integrated with their litter into groups in larger multi-suckling pens between 10–21 days post-farrowing.

Alternatively, sows are already grouped prior to farrowing and have free access to individual nest boxes for farrowing, which may or may not be removed 7–10 days post-farrowing

Outdoor systems

Outdoors, sows and their piglets are housed individually in farrowing arks or huts (Figure 4.20), with access to individual or group paddocks. There are different ark and hut designs available.

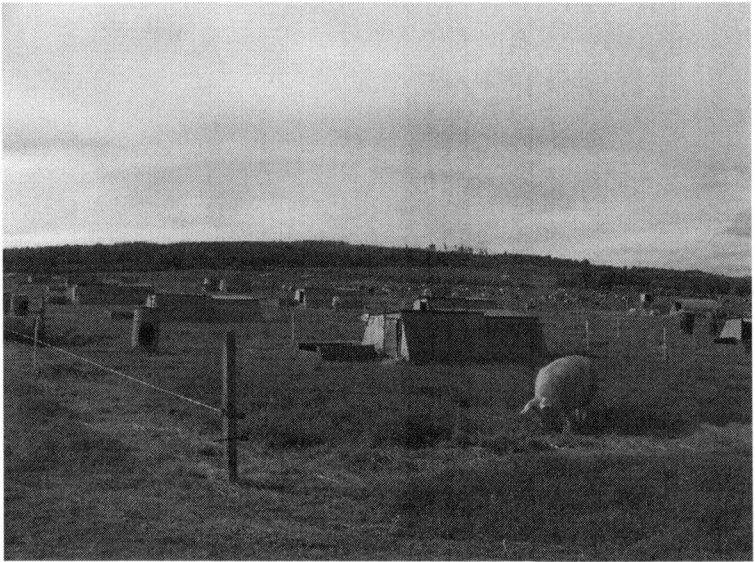

Figure 4.20 Outdoor system. Photo: SRUC / M. Farish.

4.6.3 Farrowing pain

SARAH ISON

Sow comfort is critical in the days around farrowing. The breeding sow is essential for successful production. Good sow health and welfare is reflected in her ability to produce a healthy litter of piglets: taking good care of the sow means the piglets will survive and thrive (see also Section 4.3 on piglet welfare).

For the sow, farrowing involves several challenges (Section 4.6.2). One of these is pain from uterine contractions, the delivery of piglets and resulting tissue damage in the reproductive tract. Sows must recover quickly after farrowing, gradually increasing food and water intake to produce a good supply of milk for a growing litter of piglets.

Post-partum agalactia syndrome (PPDS), which includes mastitis-metritis-agalactia (MMA) is a wide term for conditions reducing colostrum and milk production by the sow. Signs of PPDS include sows appearing lethargic, slow to feed and drink, with hungry piglets (for example, vocalizing, active at the udder). Sows may also show more subtle behaviour signs, thought

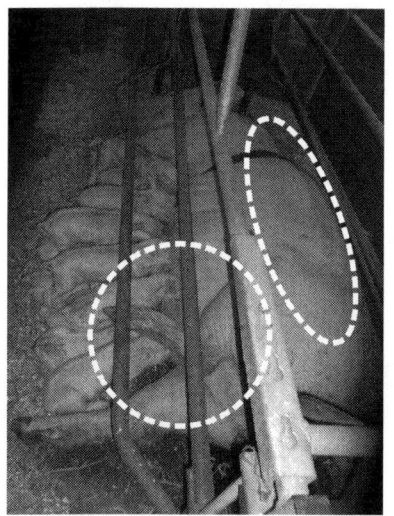

to indicate pain, like trembling, a 'hunched' (arched back) posture and pulling the back legs in towards the body (Figure 4.21). The sow may still appear to be straining as if farrowing, even when the process is complete. Routinely checking sow temperature after farrowing can also help detect early signs of PPDS enabling prompt management to reduce any negative impacts on the piglets.

Figure 4.21 A sow with an arched back posture with one back leg pulled forward. Photo: SRUC / S. Ison.

A useful addition to the management routine, especially for sows show-ing signs of PPDS or after a long and difficult farrowing, is the use of pain relief (for example, meloxicam, ketoprofen) to accelerate sow recovery. Studies testing pain relief after farrowing show multiple benefits to sow health, welfare and piglet performance, potentially leading to benefits that outweigh the cost of pain medication. Given the influence of different housing and management systems on-farm, the use of pain medication after farrowing can be evaluated using the cost–benefit analysis tool.

4.6.4 Shoulder ulcers and udder lesions

METTE S. HERSKIN AND HANNE KONGSTED

In conventional pig production systems, shoulder ulcers can be a problem in lactating sows. The term covers rounded ulcers in the skin overlying the shoulder. The lesions vary from superficial lesions, in which redness of the skin is the only clinical sign, to deep ulcers involv-ing subcutaneous layers or even bone tissue. The ulcers can be observed in the weeks after farrowing and will normally heal after the lactation period. The ulcers are to some extent comparable with human pres-sure ulcers, and develop due to pressure from the flooring and blood circulation leading to ischemic conditions and necrosis.

Shoulder ulcers can be graded pathologically, based on their depth. However, this is not easy on live sows, where instead the diameter of the lesion can be used as an indicator of the severity (Figure 4.22). Irrespectively of the size of the lesion, shoulder ulcers are a welfare problem for the affected sows. Ulcers have been shown to affect the behaviour of the sows, leading to, for example, a lower frequency of nurs-ings and more time standing idle. These effects are probably due to pain.

Not all sows develop shoulder ulcers. Sows with health problems and low body condition score are especially at risk. The early signs of shoul-der ulcers are reddening of the skin. Sows with reddened skin on the

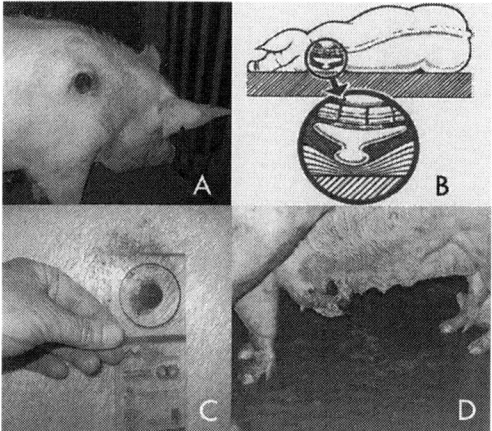

Figure 4.22 (A) A large shoulder ulcer, indicating the typical shape and localization of the lesions. (B) Schematic drawing of the situation leading to the development of shoulder ulcers: the combination of the bony prominence on the shoulder blade of sows and long periods of lying on a hard surface. (C) The diameter of shoulder ulcers is an indicator of the severity and can be monitored, for example by use of simple tools. (D) Example of udder lesion on a sow. Photos: (A) University of Copenhagen / Henrik E. Jensen; (B and C) SEGES Danish Pig Research Centre, Denmark; (D) Aarhus University / Louisa Gould.

shoulder should be offered a rubber mat or be otherwise relieved from the pressure on the shoulder area. The use of zinc ointments or similar also prevent further development of the ulcers but this is seldom effective as the sole action. Pain relief may be provided to promote healing and improve welfare. If the wound develops further, the sow must be weaned and transferred to a sick pen with softer flooring. Again, pain relief may be used. Antibiotics are seldom needed, but should be considered in advanced cases. After healing of advanced ulcers, sows should be culled in order to avoid relapse in the next lactation.

In contrast to the shoulder ulcers, udder lesions are much more heterogeneous, but still challenge the welfare of sows. Typically, udder lesions do not affect the whole udder. In contrast to shoulder ulcers, udder lesions may have several underlying causes, such as injuries inflicted by the piglets and/or bacterial infection. The pain involved in these lesions has not been documented to the same degree as for shoulder ulcers, but it is still recommended to check udders daily, stand ready to remove piglets to nurse sows and to provide pain relief.

4.7 Welfare of gestating sows

4.7.1 Pre-natal stress

WINFRIED OTTEN

Stress during gestation not only affects the welfare of sows but has also implications on growth, health and well-being of their offspring in utero and later in life. This particular form of stress is referred to as pre-natal stress. At farm level, the link between pre-natal stress and the consequences for the offspring may not be obvious, as they are different in time (next generation of animals) and location (for example, multi-site production). The gestating sow can be stressed by various adverse factors, such as restricted housing conditions, fear of humans, inadequate ambient temperatures and the social environment. Social stress during group housing of gestating sows can be caused by aggression after mixing with unfamiliar sows, by insufficient space for the avoidance of other sows or by competition at the feeding station. Studies have shown that pre-natal stress in pigs has a negative impact on growth, vitality, health and welfare of the offspring and therefore has ethical as well as economic implications.

Offspring of sows that have been stressed during gestation may show impaired growth (for example, reduced birth weight) and poor post-natal health, which may increase their mortality before weaning. In addition, behavioural abnormalities such as increased anxiety were observed later in life (Figure 4.23). This is particularly important for female offspring used for breeding, as it has been shown that sows born from pre-natally stressed mothers exhibit less maternal care. Therefore, the development

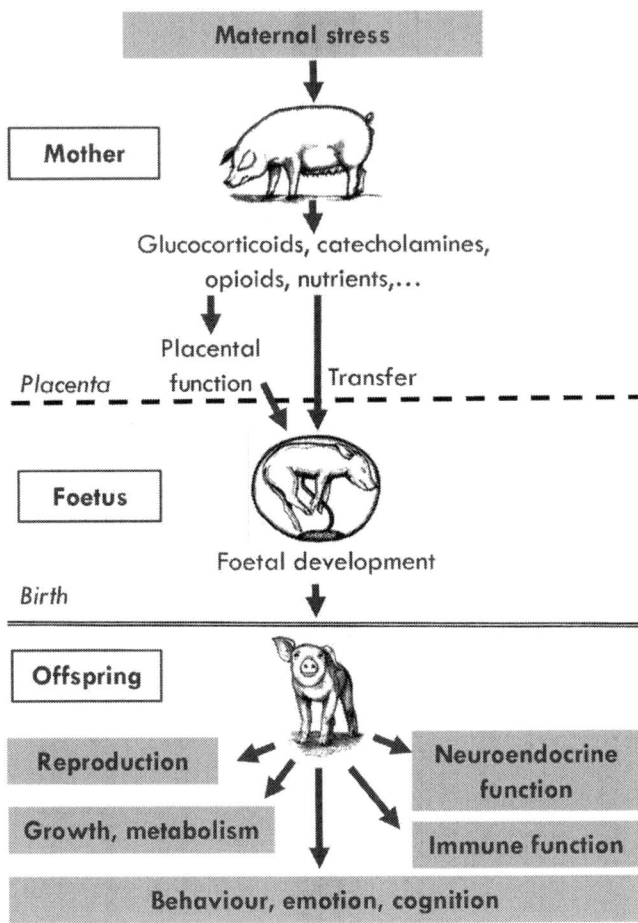

Figure 4.23 Schematic illustration of pre-natal stress and its effects on foetal development and offspring characteristics in pigs. Illustration: W. Otten.

and application of best practices for housing of gestating sows to minimize stress will improve not only the welfare of the sow but also that of its offspring with considerable economic benefits. To achieve this goal, for example, fear of humans can be mitigated by striving for positive human–animal contact and heat stress can be reduced by using evaporative cooling systems. In addition, reducing the mixing of gilts with older sows, keeping animals in familiar groups during successive gestations and providing refuge areas can reduce the negative effects of social stress during gestation on the welfare and productivity of offspring.

4.7.2 Aggression between sows

MEGAN VERDON

Sows arrange themselves into dominance hierarchies; those at the top dominate all others while those at the bottom dominate none. The intense period of aggression observed after mixing unfamiliar sows is largely due to competitive sows fighting to achieve a high rank in this hierarchy. Once the hierarchy is established it is maintained by low-ranking sows actively avoiding those more dominant. This 'active avoidance' can be difficult under commercial conditions, where space and food are often restricted. This leads to dominant sows continuing to deliver aggression even after a hierarchy has been formed. The consequences of aggression, and subsequently injuries, stress, pain and fear, make it a persistent welfare concern for group-housed sows. The intensity and duration of aggression may be minimized through effective pen design and management of sow group-housing systems (see also Section 4.4.3).

Providing sows with enough space at mixing to allow normal aggressive and submissive behaviours (avoidance), incorporating visual barriers and increasing the social experience of pigs during rearing may reduce the time and level of aggression required to form a hierarchy (as explained in Section 4.4.3). These features could be provided in a designated mixing pen while the hierarchy is established, after which sows could be moved to a smaller pen. After a hierarchy has been achieved, most of the aggression between grouped sows occurs around feeding.

Floor feeding forces low-ranking sows to risk receiving aggression by feeding in close proximity to high-ranking sows, or to avoid the area where feed is available. Individual feeding systems such as feeding stalls or electronic sow feeders offer better protection to sows while they eat, but accessing these feeders can also be competitive. A low sow to feeder ratio, long walking distance from the feeder exit to re-entry, positioning feeders away from resting or drinking spaces and maximizing total space outside of the feeder may all reduce competition for access to the feeders. High-fibre diets and foraging material may promote satiety, reducing competition and aggression at feeding (see Section 4.7.3). Other resources, for example, the drinker, foraging material, preferred lying areas, also need to be accessible to all sows.

4.7.3 Hunger

ALISTAIR B. LAWRENCE

One of the core areas of interest in the development of modern pig production has been more cost-effective feeding strategies in which feed costs are reduced without affecting performance. Feeding trials with sows in the 1980s demonstrated that litter size and quality were not affected when feed levels were reduced considerably below what sows would eat if given free choice. Hence the idea of restricted feeding regimes for sows was born and universally applied in pig production.

Restricted feeding approaches were developed entirely from the perspective of improving production. The question of how the sow perceived such a restricted diet was not considered until research suggested that restrict fed sows would remain motivated for food (would be, in other words, hungry) for much of the day. This conclusion was arrived at by training pigs to press a panel to get a small food reward to measure their motivation. Nowadays, evidence does support that modern sows are as hungry as suggested by this early work. However, questions do remain unanswered, such as whether sows are hungry when no food is on offer, as so far hunger has only been measured by offering food.

Here are some strategies to reduce the impact of restricted feeding regimes.

3 TIPS

1. Restricting food from sows might be seen as similar to controlling the weight of a pet dog or even ourselves by dieting. This comparison also suggests ways of reducing the impacts of food restriction.

2. Having control – successful dieting in humans occurs when the individual has a sense of control over the situation. Similarly allowing sows to predict accurately when they are going to be fed can successfully reduce adverse effects of hunger, such as excessive high-pitched squealing and aggression with other sows queuing for food.

3. Adding fibre can help – we know from human nutrition that adding fibre to diets can in some cases help alleviate the hunger that results from dieting. Research would suggest that fibres vary in their effectiveness in reducing hunger with one of the most effective in pigs being sugar beet pulp perhaps because of the way that sugar beet is digested.

When sows are hungry, they are motivated to forage (that is, to find food and eat it). Therefore, it is important to allow food-restricted sows space and bedding materials that allows them to express their foraging behaviour. If long straw is provided as bedding then the sows will forage in this and eat some of the straw thus allowing them some fulfilment of their motivation to search for and consume food. This solution will also often help in preventing sows from developing oral stereotypies (as described in Section 3.1.1).

4.7.4 Lameness

HELEEN A. VAN DE WEERD AND SARAH ISON

Lameness is a health issue that manifests itself as a change in the normal gait, posture and behaviour of the sow. It leads to reduced mobility from pain or discomfort, affecting sow welfare, but also the economics of a business. It can affect productivity – and therefore economics – directly (loss of animals, cost of treatment) and indirectly (via reduced production, time taken to manage lameness). As sow lameness is common, it must be identified and dealt with rapidly.

Lameness is often described as 'multifactorial'. It is influenced by multiple management variables, such as nutrition and housing (especially flooring and feeding) and group management (including mixing unfamiliar sows). Animal-related factors, such as general health and genetics (for example limb conformation), and physiological factors, such as infections of tissues, joints or bones, also play a role.

Lameness is caused by infectious or non-infectious issues with tissues (among others muscles), legs (bones, joints or cartilage) or the claws (feet) of a sow and affects her general health and behaviour (Figure 4.24). Owing to the stress and pain, the sows' immune system may be challenged or suppressed leading to an increased susceptibility to other (infectious) diseases (for example, of the urinary or reproductive tract). Lame sows may not be fit enough to compete for food and water, and this – combined with reduced activity – can increase the risk that she

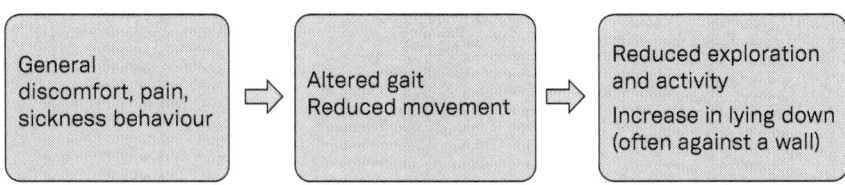

Figure 4.24 Effects of lameness on behaviour. Illustration: H.A. van de Weerd.

suffers hunger and thirst. Lameness is therefore an important (animal-based) welfare indicator (see Section 3.6).

When a lame sow is identified, the first decision is whether she can be treated (considering cost of treatment), or if euthanasia is preferred to relieve suffering. Infected claw lesions and arthritis are mainly detected in the chronic stage and prognosis is often poor. Mildly lame sows can be treated in their groups, severely lame sows are better removed to sick pens for treatment and recovery. Treatment options include the provision of pain relief (infectious and non-infectious causes), antibiotics (infectious causes) and preventative claw trimming. The best strategy is to minimize the risks of lameness (Table 4.4). Treatment and management of lameness are best discussed with the veterinarian to provide herd specific advice.

Table 4.4 Managing the risks of lameness in sows.

Aim	Strategy/action	Section
Minimize aggression at sow group formation	Space, mixing pen, enrichment	4.4.3 4.7.2
Reduce competition and aggression	Optimal pen layout (lying areas, flooring, bedding, enrichment)	4.2
Minimize competition over food	Optimal feeding systems	4.7.3
Good leg/feet conformation	Good genetics	4.9
Good bone and claw health	Optimal nutrition (vitamins and minerals), claw trimming	n/a

4.8 Welfare of cull sows

METTE S. HERSKIN

The term 'cull sow' covers the last part of the production cycle – from when the farmer decides to remove a sow and until she is dead. Cull sow management differs markedly between countries. Typically, the cull period consists of a stay in the herd (hours to weeks), transport (eventually passing buying stations or similar) and lairage at the abattoir. The majority of sows are culled due to reproductive problems or reduced productivity. At this stage, their clinical condition may be affected, as indicated by, for example, lameness, shoulder ulcers or other types of lesions.

Many sows are culled after weaning. For some days, these sows will continue to produce milk and thus maintain a high metabolism. Before transport to slaughter, cull sows are often mixed in pens on the farm of origin (Figure 4.25). The combination of continued milk production, higher metabolism and mixing is a challenge to the welfare of the sows. Upon mixing, sows will fight to establish a hierarchy. The severity of fights is increased by limited resources in the cull sow pens, such as

Figure 4.25 Newly weaned sows waiting to be picked up for slaughter, showing examples of shoulder ulcers and engorged udders. Photo: Aarhus University / Louisa Gould.

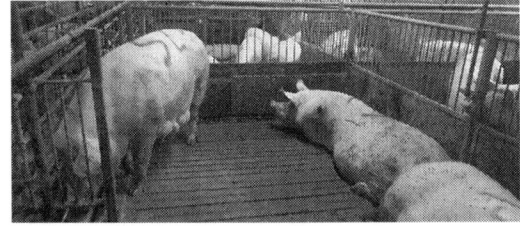

less than one feeding space per sow, restricted feeding (compared to the very high rations provided in the last part of lactation), lack of hiding space and high temperatures. Newly weaned sows are more vulnerable to heat stress due to their higher metabolism than non-lactating sows. Taken together, the mixing of cull sows is a challenge to their health and welfare.

Internationally, the number of abattoirs has decreased, which means that sows often need to travel longer journeys to slaughter than finishers. Hence, the condition of cull sows – and the conditions offered to them – is crucial for their fitness for transport. At present, only a few science-based recommendations are available for this group of animals. However, their general vulnerability combined with the tendency of sows to fight when mixed, can be a challenge during the last phase of their life – on-farm, during transport and in lairage at the abattoir. The better conditions offered to them, and the better condition they are in, the more likely it is that they will reach the abattoir successfully. If in doubt about the condition of a cull sow and her fitness for transport, consult a veterinarian for advice. And, be aware that the condition may deteriorate during transport.

4.9 Rearing gilts for a better future herd

MARTYNA M. MAŁOPOLSKA AND RYSZARD TUZ

Gilt selection and rearing are some of the most challenging, uncertain and important aspects of pig production. Good replacement gilts are a guarantee of stable production and improvement in the herd. Both animal (genetic) and environmental factors, such as feeding and housing, need to be improved. Even the best genotype will not achieve the expected results in poor environmental conditions.

Proper herd management requires systematic gilt evaluation for both reproductive and structural soundness, as these features influence future reproduction efficiency and sow-culling strategy. The prediction of reproduction ability should be based on phenotypic production traits and gilts' growth and development. Routine selection is the best method to breed the ideal gilts, thus pre-selection should begin with careful matching of sire and dam with high reproduction efficiency, and maternal ability. Then, gilts should be selected on the day of weaning, choosing more gilts as needed as replacements. This will reduce the risk and give a wide range of comparison and selection between females. The decision should be based on the health of individuals, pre-weaning average daily gain and body weight at weaning (at least 7.5 kg). From this time gilts should be reared separately from the rest of the offspring, on appropriate space with access to environmental enrichment materials, such as toys. Visual evaluation of structure should be made at around 140 days of age, with respect to feet, legs, underline, external genitalia, body weight, body condition, backfat thickness and growth rate. It is important to focus on as many traits as possible to increase the effectiveness of prediction. It can make it easier to divide the selection criteria into categories.

Criterion 1: structural soundness and condition – focusing on hooves, legs (strong, straight, set to pasterns, wide apart) and locomotion, body weight and backfat thickness. Gilts characterized by 16–17 mm of backfat thickness are more likely to achieve large, heavy litters. Condition during pregnancy and reduced piglet crushing risk during farrowing are positively affected by properly developed limbs. Maintaining an appropriate body weight during lactation protects females against excessive weight loss.

Criterion 2: reproductive organs – udder (number of functional nipples, size, shape, location) and vulva (well developed, well shaped, proportional in size, tip pointing downward). Gilts should have at least 14 to 16 well developed nipples, in a straight line.

Criterion 3: body weight and litter size at birth – dam's fertility, milk production, reproductive history (in the same housing conditions of dam, the performance of the female offspring of dam and her siblings) and maternal ability (behavioural observations of each individual) are good sources of information. Choosing gilts based on litter size has two main methods: from the largest, heaviest litter and from smaller litters. Both have advantages and disadvantages, so observations and even comparison of these two methods, in particular herds, is necessary to decide which method will give better results. Following the first method (based on largest litter), dams should have at least 12–13 piglets and a high fertility rate, which should be calculated on reproduction data for three parities. The second method is based on smaller litters, and here gilts have more uterine space and so better conditions for development and growth in pre- and post-natal environments. Moreover, the composition of sexes in litter is also important. Large number of boars (> 60%) can cause problems with gilts' reproduction from this litter, as well as with the number of their nipples. The preponderance of males reduces number of nipples in gilts from such litters.

Criterion 4: growth rates – gilts should not exceed 700 g/day, which is a natural protection against overweight and ensures proper development of the reproductive tract. Additionally, a rapid uncontrolled growth can lead to production issues, such as small litter size. Reproduction issues are the main reason for culling sows in early parities from a breeding herd. Consequently, frequent replacement of females can lower herd productivity and causes interruption in social hierarchy.

When gilts reached between 90–100 kg, they should be exposed to boar stimulation. After stimulation gilts achieve first oestrus sooner, have more piglets in their first litter and consequently their lifetime productivity will be greater. The first oestrus is a sign off onset of puberty in gilts. Age of first oestrus and then the time of mating or insemination have an impact on subsequent reproductive performance and sow longevity. Many factors influenced the age of puberty, including genotype, technique and effectiveness of oestrus detection, season, environment, boar exposure, nutrition and health. Usually, sexual maturity occurs at 180 to 210 days, but in colder climates this time could be delayed, even to 270 days. It is worth mentioning that rapid development of the reproductive tract starts at 6 months of age (first oestrus), so to prevent gilts from negative effects and small numbers of offspring, it is recommended to mate gilts at second or even third oestrus.

An additional tool that indicates reproductive efficiency is the measurement (with use of AI catheter during first oestrus) of vaginal and cervical length (VCL), which reflects uterine capacity. Simultaneously with an increase in uterine size the number of piglets obtained increases. Also, more available uterine space reduces pre-natal mortality and supports good foetal growth. Owing to the great diversity of VCL between females, breeds and lines, it is necessary to conduct routine measurement and monitor reproduction data and maternal responsiveness for each animal. This long-term method is beneficial and gives detailed data of each female in the herd.

To obtain the best reproductive efficiency from gilts a combination of traditional selection should be used with increased selection intensity and the addition of new methods, based on maternal responsiveness (sensitivity) and VCL measurements. Successful gilt rearing depends on proper environmental conditions (housing system, feeding, temperature and so on), genotype and proper selection of replacement gilts. All the above factors affect sow longevity and decrease culling rates, which improve both herd and individual welfare.

 **4.10** Make a stepwise action plan for improving welfare

We have given you many recommendations to improve the welfare of pigs in practice. The table on the next page provides a checklist for each topic with the main factor(s) to consider. If you have staff, each staff member should fill in the list and the lists can then be compared. It is good to discuss these topics and come to an agreement on which aspects can be improved and the priority that should be given to each aspect. In the second table suggestions to improve the aspects are provided.

Topic	Question	Yes	Can be better	No	Priority yes/no
Human–animal interaction	Are the pigs calm and can be handled efficiently?				
Enrichment	Is enrichment available?				
	Is the enrichment suitable for the age/type of animal?				
	Is the enrichment in the correct place?				
Neonatal piglets	Is the mortality reasonable given the litter size?				
	Can the sows nurse their piglets well?				
Procedures	Is pain relief/anaesthesia given when castrating?				

	Are procedures carried out quickly with minimal stress to piglets and sow?				
Euthanasia	Are the staff members proficient in performing euthanasia on piglets?				
Weaning	Does weaning provide a gradual transition of changes?				
	Does weaning stress subside after one day?				
Tail biting	Is attention paid to the tail posture?				
Aggression	Is regrouping minimized?				
Boars	Is the welfare of the boars similar to the gilts?				
Nest building	Do the sows have some form of nest building material?				
Farrowing pen	Is the farrowing pen design optimal?				
	Would the pens be suitable to transition to free farrowing pens?				
Pain relief	Is pain relief given to sows when required?				
Lying comfort	Are sows free from lying injuries?				
	Can sows stand up easily in the pen?				
Prenatal stress	Is stress minimized during gestation?				
Sow aggression	Is regrouping of sows largely avoided?				
Hunger	Are sows fed roughage?				
Cull sows	Are cull sows in reasonable condition when transported?				
Gilt rearing	Are the gilts calm and used to human contact?				

If you answered 'No' or 'Can be better' in these questions and the topic is of relevance to the farm then it is recommended to look into the respective chapters. The main recommendations from Chapter 4 are given here.

Topic	Suggestion
Human–animal interaction	Improve human–animal interaction by frequent calm (hand) contact and using a calm voice. Give the pigs more positive experiences with humans.
Enrichment	Provide enrichment appropriate to the age and type of pig.
	Ensure that materials are chewable, edible, deformable, can be used together, and do not pose a risk.
	Adjust the enrichment to the right height and ensure that it does not get soiled.
Neonatal piglets	Do not push the genetics for large litter size if the housing and management available is not suitable for it.
	Select the right genetics to optimize number and vitality of weaned piglets within the system.
Procedures	Consider options that minimize pain.
	Think of how procedures can be done more efficiently, for example, by treating piglets in a separate room.
Euthanasia	Provide staff training on best practice.
Weaning	Consider spreading the stressful events for pigs over several days by removing the sow before moving piglets.
	Aim to keep litters together to minimize aggression. Make weaning as smooth as possible.
Tail biting	Train staff to pay attention to tail posture to detect tail biting early on. Use the action plan in Section 4.4.2 for further steps.
Aggression	Minimize regrouping when possible.
Boars	House boars with appropriate flooring to reduce lameness due to mounting.
Nest building	Provide some form of nest material to reduce sow stress, even if just a few handfuls of hay/straw.
Farrowing pen	See if small things can be improved at reasonable costs.
	If the farm is in Europe, think ahead for the possibility that free farrowing might be a new standard in the future.

Pain relief	Consider giving pain relief when sows have difficulty with farrowing.
Lying comfort	Provide mats or different flooring to reduce injuries.
	Consider adjusting the roughness of the floor or a bar to stand/lie more easily.
Pre-natal stress	Assess stressful situations for pregnant sows and discuss how these can be minimized. Look at improving handling, and of minimizing heat stress due to increasing environmental temperatures.
Sow aggression	Aim to keep stable groups of sows and introduce new sows gradually. Interfere when needed.
Hunger	Provide roughage or foraging materials for sows.
Cull sows	Provide cull sows with a comfortable pen with bedding to gain energy/recover ahead of transport. Avoid regrouping of weak sows.
Gilt rearing	Have daily contact with the gilts, using voice and touch.

Appendices

Appendix 1: Welfare Quality® form for sows and piglets

Principle		Welfare criteria	Measures
Good feeding	1	Absence of prolonged hunger	**Sow (S):** Body condition **Piglet (P):** Age of weaning
	2	Absence of prolonged thirst	**S, P:** Water supply
Good housing	3	Comfort around resting	**S:** Bursitis, shoulder sores **S, P:** Absence of manure on the body
	4	Thermal comfort	**S, P:** Panting, huddling
	5	Ease of movement	**S:** Space allowance, farrowing crates
Good health	6	Absence of injuries	**S, P:** Lameness **S:** Wounds on the body, vulva lesions
	7	Absence of disease	**S, P:** Mortality, coughing, sneezing, pumping, rectal prolapse, scouring **S:** Constipation, metritis, mastitis, uterine prolapse, skin condition, hernias, local infections **P:** Neurological disorders, splay leg
	8	Absence of pain induced by management procedures	**S:** Nose ringing and tail docking **P:** Castration, tail docking and teeth clipping
Appropriate behaviour	9	Expression of social behaviours	**S:** Social behaviour
	10	Expression of other behaviours	**S:** Stereotypies, exploratory behaviour
	11	Human–animal relationship	**S:** Fear of humans
	12	Positive emotional state	**S, P:** Qualitative Behaviour Assessment (QBA)

Appendix 2: Welfare Quality® form for growing pigs

Principle		Welfare criteria	Measures
Good feeding	1	Absence of prolonged hunger	Body condition score
	2	Absence of prolonged thirst	Water supply
Good housing	3	Comfort around resting	Bursitis, absence of manure on the body
	4	Thermal comfort	Shivering, panting, huddling
	5	Ease of movement	Space allowance
Good health	6	Absence of injuries	Lameness, wounds on the body, tail biting
	7	Absence of disease	Mortality, coughing, sneezing, pumping, twisted snouts, rectal prolapse, scouring, skin condition, hernias
	8	Absence of pain induced by management procedures	Castration, tail docking
Appropriate behaviour	9	Expression of social behaviours	Social behaviour
	10	Expression of other behaviours	Exploratory behaviour
	11	Good human–animal relationship	Fear of humans
	12	Positive emotional state	Qualitative Behaviour Assessment (QBA)

Appendix 3: Scoring list for pig qualitative behaviour assessment

Active

Min   Max

Relaxed

Min   Max

Fearful

Min   Max

Agitated

Min   Max

Calm

Min   Max

Content

Min   Max

Tense

Min   Max

Enjoying

Min   Max

Frustrated

Min   Max

Sociable

Min   Max

Bored

Min — Max

Aimless

Min — Max

Playful

Min — Max

Positively
Occupied

Min — Max

Listless

Min — Max

Lively

Min — Max

Indifferent

Min — Max

Irritable

Min — Max

Aimless

Min — Max

Happy

Min — Max

Distressed

Min — Max

Appendix 4: Checklists for suitability of enrichment objects

Guidance: describe the object to score. Use – / + / + + and % (for pig in pen). Rank the objects from optimal, suboptimal to marginal (least effective). If only suboptimal objects are available, combine to enhance characteristics.

Object	Object characteristics				
	Investigable (rootable)	Manipulable	Chewable (deformable)	Destructible	Edible
[describe object]	[score]	[score]	[score]	[score]	[score]

	Method of provision	
Object	Able to sustain interest?	Accessible to how many pigs simultaneously? (0–100%)
[describe object]	[score]	[% of pigs in pen]

Appendix 5: Calculation guide for the amount of enrichment material

1. Choose a moment in the day when the majority of pigs are active and not eating or sleeping.

2. Count the number of pigs that are exploring (manipulating, investigating, chewing) enrichment material. This figure corresponds to 'A'.

3. Count the number of pigs interacting with other pigs and pen fittings (do not include eating and drinking). This figure corresponds to 'B'.

4. Substitute the letters in this equation with your figures:

    $$\text{Amount needed} = (A/A+B) * 100$$

5. Example: if 20 pigs are exploring the enrichment material, with an additional 10 pigs interacting with other pigs or fittings, the sum would be 20/30. Now multiply that answer by 100 to give you a percentage (in this case: 66.7%).

6. Compare your figures with these categories

    -   0–18% Minimal exploratory behaviour – introduction of enrichment materials is recommended.
    -   18.1–86% Intermediate exploratory behaviour – no additional material required, but consider providing more if the figure is close to the lower end of the range.
    -   86.1–100% Maximum exploratory behaviour – no additional material required.

This information is derived from the European Commission leaflet 'Cutting the need for tail docking' (available in Danish, Dutch, English, French, German, Spanish, Italian, Polish, https://ec.europa.eu/food/animals/welfare/practice/farm/pigs/tail-docking_en).

Index